Quinoa

HIGH PROTEIN, GLUTEN-FREE

Beth Geisler

with recipes by Jo Stepaniak

books
Alive
Summertown
TENNESSEE

CONTENTS

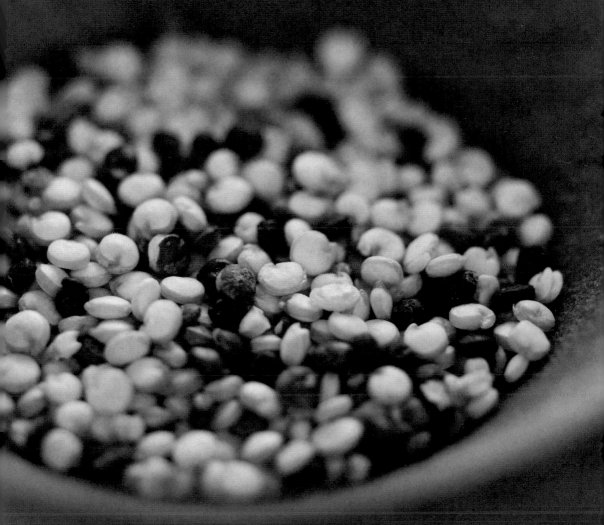

quinoa
HIGH PROTEIN, GLUTEN-FREE

*Quinoa (KEEN-wah) is technically a seed,
although it's often called a grain.*

INTRODUCING QUINOA

In North America, the conversation about quinoa, an ancient grain from South America, started in the 1980s when it was first imported. And it's been heating up ever since. That's because this nutritious food is high in protein, has an outstanding amino acid profile, is lower in carbohydrates than other whole grains, and is rich in minerals and vitamins. These, among other nutrition advantages, have earned quinoa the nicknames "superfood" and "supergrain."

Quinoa's flavor, often described as nutty, is mellow and comforting, and its texture is fluffy and sometimes a bit crunchy depending on the type of quinoa and how well it's been cooked. Light and easy to digest, the grain is exceptionally versatile and can provide endless variety in any cook's repertoire. It can be substituted for almost any other grain, such as rice, couscous, barley, millet, and bulgur. It can also be an alternative to pasta and potatoes. Commercially, quinoa is available in many forms, including cold breakfast cereals, flakes, flour, and gluten-free pasta.

The first task for a person who is new to quinoa is to learn how to properly say the name—the word is pronounced KEEN-wah. The next is to discover all the reasons this superfood is cropping up all over. Now widely available in natural food stores, supermarkets, and online outlets, quinoa meets the needs of consumers who seek an organically grown, hypoallergenic, gluten-free whole grain. These attributes mean that quinoa is unlikely to trigger food allergies and is suitable for people who can't eat wheat or other cereal grains.

Quinoa is exported mostly from Bolivia and Peru, where it's still sustainably grown by farming families and is sown by hand, weeded by hand, harvested by hand, and threshed by hand. A number of brands on the market are fair-trade products, available in North America through the collaboration of farmers, farming collectives, and selective importers.

Considered to be a nutritionally complete plant-based food, quinoa has been a favorite among vegetarians and vegans for some time. But it has quickly moved into the mainstream, and savvy cooks everywhere are introducing it

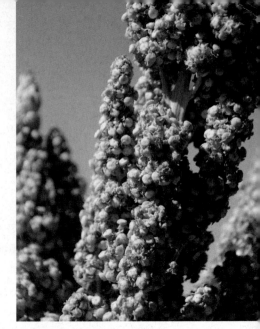

to their friends and families. As its popularity grows, quinoa is gaining attention, and not just at dinner parties. This nutritious crop has been noticed by organizations that recognize its potential for the future. For example, the United Nations sees it as a crop that could alleviate hunger and malnutrition because it can be grown in arid regions where other crops won't survive. In addition, the National Aeronautics and Space Administration (NASA) has studied quinoa as a food source that could be grown on long-term manned space flights, providing nutrition and sustenance to the crew.

A Seed, Not a True Grain

Technically, quinoa (*Chenopodium quinoa*) is not a true grain but the seed of a plant in the goosefoot family. Its relatives include not only common food crops, such as beets, chard, and spinach, but also wild plants, such as lamb's-quarters, which grows abundantly throughout North America. As a seed crop, quinoa, like amaranth and buckwheat, is sometimes referred to as a "pseudograin" or "pseudocereal" because it's used like a grain and is nutritionally similar. Often, however, quinoa is simply called a grain, and that's the term used throughout this book.

Most grains, such as wheat, oats, barley, and rye, come from plants that are members of the grass species. And just like grains from the grass family, quinoa can be easily ground into flour. Grains and pseudograins are excellent sources of energy and protein. In fact, quinoa has up to twice the amount of protein as many grains.

Flat, irregularly shaped, and quite small, quinoa seeds are about the size of millet or sesame seeds. A close look will reveal the reason for the seeds' unusual shape—like all whole grains, quinoa has a germ. This tail-like germ protrudes slightly in the dry grain; when cooked in liquid, the germ curls around the grain like a tiny halo.

Quinoa seeds grow in large clusters at the top of the plant's tall, magenta stalk, and a field planted with quinoa can reveal a riot of brilliant color. The flowering plant can feature blossoms that range from crimson to orange to violet, and the seed heads can be green, orange, pink, purple, red, or yellow. Once the seed head is dried, the tiny quinoa seeds are simply shaken out and dried. The next step removes some of the seeds' brilliant color, which is caused by a natural resin that acts as the plants' own defense system against birds and insects that would feast on the seeds. Because of this natural resinous coating, quinoa can be grown without chemical pesticides. The resin, which may even protect the seeds from the extreme heat they're exposed to at high altitudes, contains 2 to 6 percent saponin, a mild toxin that produces a soapy lather. When the resin is removed from the quinoa, the color may also be stripped away, leaving the white, red, and black quinoa varieties that are sold commercially.

The saponin-containing resin causes quinoa to taste bitter, and most growers remove it either by soaking the seeds in water or by using machinery similar to a rice polisher. Nonetheless, although many brands say they're prerinsed, quinoa should always be soaked or rinsed before cooking to avoid potential bitterness. The cooking technique recommended in this book includes a brief soaking, which helps to remove any residual saponin. After the quinoa has been soaked, simply put it in a fine-mesh strainer and thoroughly rinse it for a few moments to ensure that any saponin has been removed; that will be evident when the rinse water no longer foams or produces lather.

In South America, the saponin that is removed after harvest has traditionally been used as a shampoo, a detergent for clothing, and an antiseptic for wounds. Some farmers have even found that the saponin-laced water that remains after quinoa has been washed is an effective fertilizer. When saponin is removed by mechanical means, such as polishing, the resulting powder is used in soaps, detergents, cosmetics, pharmaceuticals, and other applications.

Read on for more information about quinoa's ancient history in South America and its promise for the future, its role as a nutrition powerhouse and gluten-free food, and how to use it in the kitchen in a variety of savory and sweet dishes. For recipes to get you acquainted with using quinoa, see pages 42 to 58.

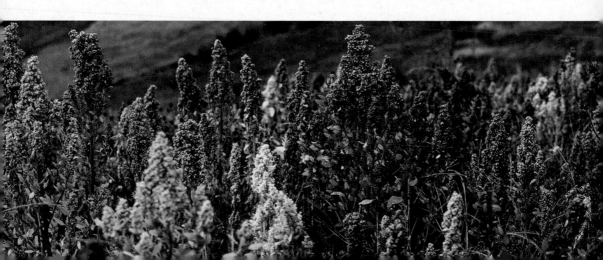

QUINOA'S PAST AND PROMISE

Since 3000 BC in South America, the indigenous people of the Andean Altiplano (see sidebar, page 8) cultivated quinoa and relied upon it as a staple food. They called it *chisiya mama*, or "mother grain." By the time the Incas rose to power in the fifteenth century, an annual ceremony marked the significance of the sacred grain. In a kingly act, the Incan emperor himself planted the first seeds of the year using a golden spade. All too soon, however, the Inca's very short reign was nearing its end, and quinoa's long supremacy was also in jeopardy.

In just one year, between 1532 and 1533, the Spanish conquered the Inca Empire, destroying the quinoa fields and forbidding further cultivation. They dismissed the grain as peasant food. In remote areas, locals continued to grow quinoa in keeping with ancient traditions. The invaders' scorn was pervasive, however, and over time quinoa fell out of favor among the indigenous people, who also came to regard it as inferior. Despite the end of colonial rule in the 1800s, when it was no longer illegal to grow quinoa, enthusiasm for the crop waned. Still, cultivation continued, and quinoa began to draw the interest of outsiders. Periodically, North Americans and Europeans who had visited the Andes published their findings about this intriguing crop, but quinoa's "rediscovery" had yet to occur.

Three North Americans, David Cusack, Stephen Gorad, and Don McKinley, are credited with introducing quinoa to the United States in the 1980s after discovering it in Bolivia. They imported the grain, and it was on supermarket shelves by 1988. Around the same time, these early quinoa pioneers and their associates grew the crop successfully in Colorado. In the ensuing decades, people everywhere got the news about this superfood, and demand for it grew. In South America, small-scale farmers and their associations, or cooperatives, prospered as they grew the crop for export, and indigenous people once again embraced the grain in their own diets. Quinoa cultivation was on the rise.

Indeed, quinoa has had a fascinating past. But the more interesting story may ultimately be its promise for the future. Organizations such as the United Nations (UN) view quinoa as a sustainable solution for hunger across the globe. In fact, the UN calls quinoa the "ancestral gift from the Andes to the world." That's a huge journey for such a tiny grain, but it doesn't stop there.

THE ANDEAN ALTIPLANO

Quinoa is grown primarily on the Altiplano in the Andes mountain range in west-central South America. The Altiplano is a high plains region that lies at an altitude between 12,000 feet (about 3,500 meters) and 14,000 feet (about 4,300 meters). The vast, cold, windswept, and barren plateau spans Bolivia and Peru, including Lake Titicaca, along with parts of Argentina and Chile.

You might think that a crop that grows at altitudes of 13,000 feet on the world's second-tallest plateau couldn't reach much greater heights, but the National Aeronautics and Space Administration (NASA) would disagree. Research has found quinoa to be a viable crop to cultivate in space during long-term manned space flights. Read on for the details that could take quinoa from the ancient Andes to the final frontier.

Early History

Agricultural practices began to emerge in the Andean Altiplano between 8000 and 7000 BC. The indigenous people likely started transforming quinoa from a wild plant to a cultivated crop between 5,000 and 7,000 years ago. While there is some archaeological evidence that domesticated seeds may have existed nearly 8,000 years ago (see sidebar, page 9), today most historians say quinoa has been cultivated in the Altiplano since 3000 BC.

The evolution of wild camelids, the ancestors of today's alpacas and llamas, appears to be tied to that of quinoa. It's likely that people began to pay attention to quinoa's potential as a food crop after the wild form was used as fodder for the animals, and the farmers manipulated the

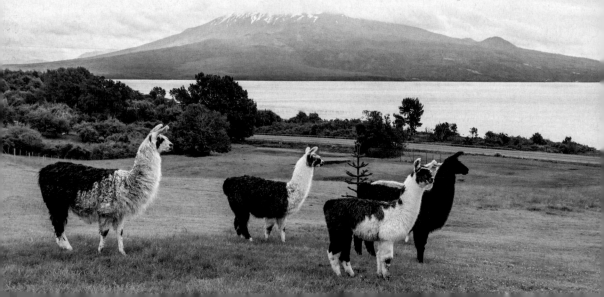

AN ANCIENT CROP

Archaeologists found what may be the earliest domestic quinoa seeds in cave deposits in the Ayacucho basin of Peru. Based on interpretations of the rock strata, the seeds could be up to 7,800 years old, but other types of testing couldn't confirm this timeline. Additional research has shown that quinoa found in a cave site in Panalauca, also in Peru, originated up to 4,000 years ago.

crop to become a good food source for both animals and humans. A mutually beneficial relationship existed between the camelids, quinoa, and people for centuries. The crop provided food, and the animals provided labor and fertilizer. To this day llama manure is used as an organic fertilizer to regenerate the soil where quinoa is grown. However, as more land is being used for crops and less for animal herding, fewer animals means a shortage of this traditional fertilizer.

For centuries, quinoa and other Andean crops were grown in raised field systems. This method of agricultural production used elevated planting platforms that were narrow and long. A portion of the land was planted, but much of the valuable space was dedicated to canal systems that directed seasonal rainfall, natural springs, groundwater, and other irrigation sources. These raised field and terraced systems of early societies aren't quite as prevalent in the Andean highlands today, although crops are still planted on flat terraces.

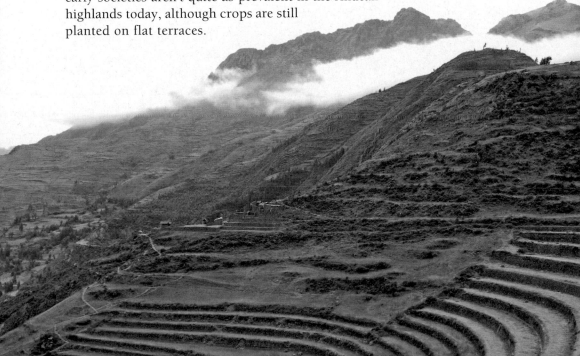

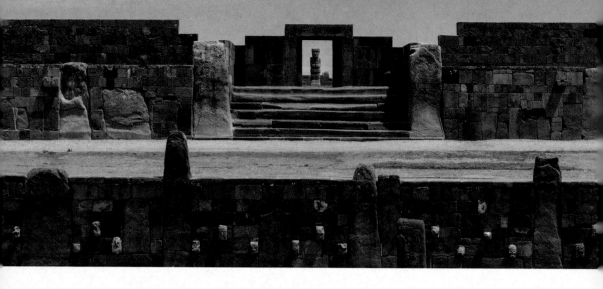

The Aymara, Incas, and Spanish

The Aymara, an Indian people who have existed for more than ten thousand years, have cultivated quinoa for thousands of years. Long predating the Incas, the Aymara were a great advanced civilization in their own right. They started to grow crops around Lake Titicaca after 4000 BC, and by 600 AD they had built a vast city on the lakeshore. That grand city, Tiahuanaco, featured immense stone structures, including pyramids and temples, but was abandoned about 1100 AD, possibly because of drought.

Today the way of life for many rural Aymara is quite similar to that of their long-ago ancestors. Holding fast to their traditions, they continue to make a living by herding and farming, and quinoa still features prominently in their culture.

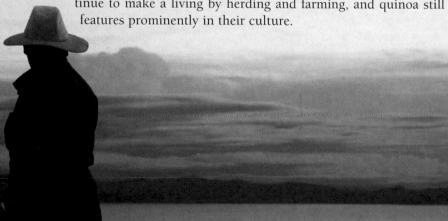

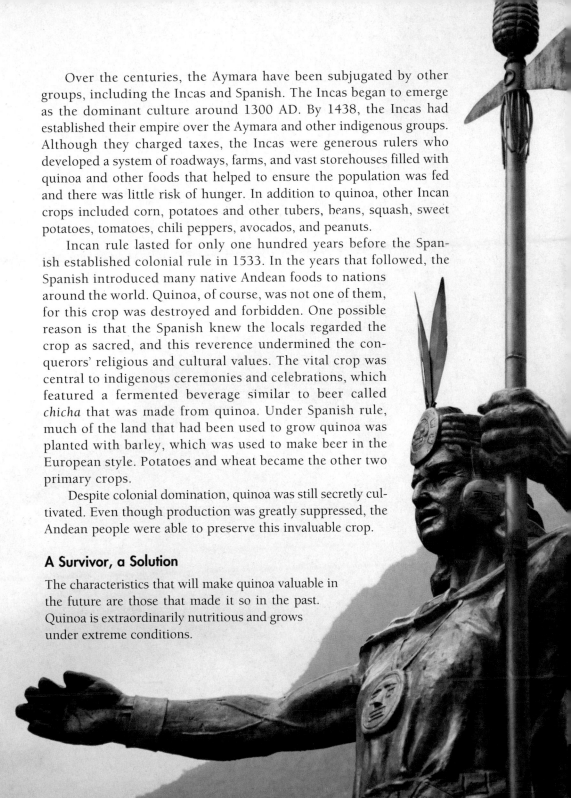

Over the centuries, the Aymara have been subjugated by other groups, including the Incas and Spanish. The Incas began to emerge as the dominant culture around 1300 AD. By 1438, the Incas had established their empire over the Aymara and other indigenous groups. Although they charged taxes, the Incas were generous rulers who developed a system of roadways, farms, and vast storehouses filled with quinoa and other foods that helped to ensure the population was fed and there was little risk of hunger. In addition to quinoa, other Incan crops included corn, potatoes and other tubers, beans, squash, sweet potatoes, tomatoes, chili peppers, avocados, and peanuts.

Incan rule lasted for only one hundred years before the Spanish established colonial rule in 1533. In the years that followed, the Spanish introduced many native Andean foods to nations around the world. Quinoa, of course, was not one of them, for this crop was destroyed and forbidden. One possible reason is that the Spanish knew the locals regarded the crop as sacred, and this reverence undermined the conquerors' religious and cultural values. The vital crop was central to indigenous ceremonies and celebrations, which featured a fermented beverage similar to beer called *chicha* that was made from quinoa. Under Spanish rule, much of the land that had been used to grow quinoa was planted with barley, which was used to make beer in the European style. Potatoes and wheat became the other two primary crops.

Despite colonial domination, quinoa was still secretly cultivated. Even though production was greatly suppressed, the Andean people were able to preserve this invaluable crop.

A Survivor, a Solution

The characteristics that will make quinoa valuable in the future are those that made it so in the past. Quinoa is extraordinarily nutritious and grows under extreme conditions.

FOOD FIT FOR AN ARMY

The ancient Incas recognized quinoa as a highly nutritious food that was able to provide energy and improve stamina. In fact, it's well known that Inca warriors carried and ate a highly portable food referred to as "war balls," made from a mixture of fat and quinoa. Possibly the world's first energy bars, this high-protein food has gained renown for enhancing the soldiers' strength and endurance.

According to Alan Kolata, professor of anthropology and social sciences at the University of Chicago, quinoa survives exceptionally well under conditions that make it impossible for other food crops to survive. In fact, its ability to survive defines the potential importance of this grain.

Kolata's interests include agriculture and rural development, particularly in the Andean region, and he wrote a paper about the production, consumption, and social value of quinoa. His was an early voice encouraging modern agronomists not to dismiss the Altiplano as an agriculturally viable region despite its harsh environment. Kolata also emphasized the nutritional value of quinoa, acknowledging its high protein and amino acid content. In addition, he noted that the relatively high fat content of quinoa compared to other grains provides caloric value, which was essential for indigenous people.

Further addressing the crop's remarkable survival in harsh environments, he praised quinoa's ability to grow on nutrient-depleted soils in marginal areas and to flourish in the frost-prone Altiplano. In fact, some varieties of quinoa are so frost-tolerant, they're able to reproduce consistently in harsh climatic conditions. The following are some of the traits that make quinoa so resilient:

- grows at sea level or high altitudes (up to 13,000 feet or roughly 4,000 meters)
- thrives in cool temperatures but adapts to extremes, from 17 degrees F (-8 degrees C) to 100 degrees F (38 degrees C)
- grows in dry regions, requiring little water
- survives droughts that wipe out other crops
- grows in depleted and even highly saline soil
- tolerates frost
- needs no chemical pesticides because natural saponins protect the seeds

In particular, quinoa's tolerance of arid conditions makes it a candidate for planting in areas affected by desertification and land degradation caused by climate change. It's little wonder quinoa has caught the attention of the UN, which, like Kolata, recognizes this ancient crop's potential to help alleviate world hunger.

Using the theme "A future sown thousands of years ago," the UN's General Assembly declared 2013 the International Year of Quinoa in honor of the Andean indigenous people who have managed to preserve quinoa in its natural state as a food for present and future generations. The reason that quinoa may be such a pivotal crop in the future is because it can grow in areas where global climate change has limited the ability of other cops to grow. Quinoa has adapted to environmental conditions created by the industrialized world. Specifically, it can survive in climatic and meteorological extremes. In fact, it not only survives but also thrives under conditions of drought, which are becoming more common.

The UN acknowledges that if quinoa were produced on a much larger scale in the future, it could provide food security for the world's poor and hungry in the next century. According to the US Department of Agriculture, "food security" refers to a household's economic and social conditions that ensure sufficient access to food.

Furthermore, the UN acknowledges quinoa's value as a vegetable protein that could be substituted for animal protein. Such a shift would have substantial positive effects on the environment in addition to public health if the consumption of beef and other meats were reduced. Here are some eye-opening facts that were released by the UN in 2006 that demonstrate just how substantially animal agriculture affects the environment: cattle rearing generates more global-warming greenhouse gases than driving cars. Cattle rearing also is a major source of land and water degradation. In fact, the livestock business is one of the greatest sources of pollution to the earth's increasingly scarce water sources, contributing animal wastes, antibiotics, hormones, and chemicals. This destruction is alleviated whenever people opt for plant-based foods, like protein-rich quinoa, over animal protein.

Cultivation of quinoa has expanded to include Europe, India, Kenya, and North America, although most of the crop is still farmed through traditional means in the Andean Altiplano. According to the UN, countries that are involved in agronomic trials and are exploring the commercial production of quinoa include Canada, China, Denmark, Italy, Morocco, and the Netherlands.

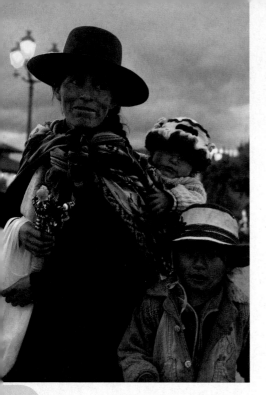

Economic Factors

Most of the world's quinoa is still grown on the Altiplano, where hundreds of thousands of small-scale farmers and their associations, or cooperatives, use sustainable practices and typically harvest the crop manually. The crop's increasing international popularity promises improved income for these farmers. One troubling factor, however, is that as prices for quinoa rise in line with demand, growers may be tempted to sell the crop and eat cheaper, less nutritious foods themselves. Some farming cooperatives try to prevent this situation by requiring the farmers to retain a portion (such as 10 to 30 percent) of their quinoa crops to feed their families.

For the most part, however, quinoa's growing popularity worldwide has led to a rediscovery of this food back home, where it has once again become a staple. Research has shown that childhood malnutrition has dropped dramatically in areas where quinoa is being grown. For example, one study showed that malnutrition dropped from 74 percent in 1998 to 20 percent in 2008 among children who live in areas where quinoa is cultivated. In addition, to combat early malnutrition, governments are advocating the food for mothers and children. As part of a nutritional supplement program, Bolivia supplies quinoa to pregnant and nursing women, and Peru incorporates quinoa in school breakfasts. But like others in developing areas, Andeans have increased access to nontraditional products, such as sodas, which the younger generation prefers over homemade quinoa drinks, and many aren't consuming as much nutritious quinoa as their long-ago ancestors.

Within the Altiplano, most quinoa is grown in Bolivia and Peru. The UN's Food and Agricultural Organization reports that these countries account for more than half of the 70,000 tons of quinoa produced annually, with the United States responsible for about 7,000 tons. Furthermore, the organization estimates that in 2003, quinoa sold for less than $70 per ton, and by 2013 that price had risen to $2,000. Roncagliolo Orbegoso, Peru's minister of foreign affairs, points out that in 2012, his country exported over $30 million worth of quinoa to thirty-seven markets abroad, including Australia, Canada, Germany, Israel, and the United States.

QUINOA IS ALSO A VEGETABLE

Quinoa leaves—like the leaves of its relatives, beets, chard, and spinach—are edible and highly nutritious greens. The leaves can be served raw in salads or added to hot dishes, such as soups and stews. Especially rich in vitamin A, quinoa leaves are consumed where the crop is grown; unfortunately, however, the green hasn't yet become commercially available in North America despite the fact that NASA recognizes the value of this healthy food for space travelers.

The United States and Beyond

In the United States, quinoa was virtually unknown before the 1980s, when Stephen Gorad and Don McKinley founded the Quinoa Corporation after bringing the first fifty-pound bag of the grain into the country. Initially, Gorad and McKinley imported quinoa for sale in natural food stores, where it was available by 1984, and then in supermarkets, where it was available by 1988. With David Cusack, other associates, and Colorado State University, they also set out to grow quinoa in Colorado's San Luis Valley, which features farming conditions similar to those in the Andean Altiplano. The first commercial quinoa crop of 100,000 pounds was harvested in 1987. Today, the Quinoa Corporation sells its products under the Ancient Harvest brand (see Resources, page 60).

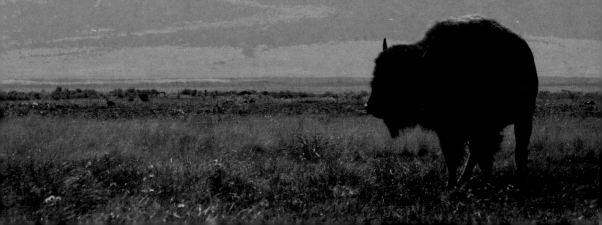

It wasn't long before the rocket scientists took notice. Since the 1990s, NASA has researched quinoa for its Controlled Ecological Life Support System (CELSS). Quinoa ranks high on the list of potential foods for long-term space missions, which could last for years. One goal of CELSS is to use plants to remove carbon dioxide from the atmosphere of a ship or space station and to generate food and oxygen for crew members.

Quinoa is an outstanding candidate for space travel because of its high productivity and nutritional characteristics, particularly its high protein level, which was nearly 21 percent in NASA's controlled growing conditions, as compared to the average crop, which is around 16 percent. A unique advantage is that the crop provides both an edible leafy vegetable and a grain (see sidebar, page 15). Even the saponins, which can be used to produce soaps, detergents, shampoos, and pharmaceuticals, may be beneficial in space.

All of these nods to quinoa's space-age potential are well deserved, but one additional fact is also worth remembering. Wherever it's used, this versatile grain can be incorporated into virtually any cuisine with the same result: the taste is out of this world.

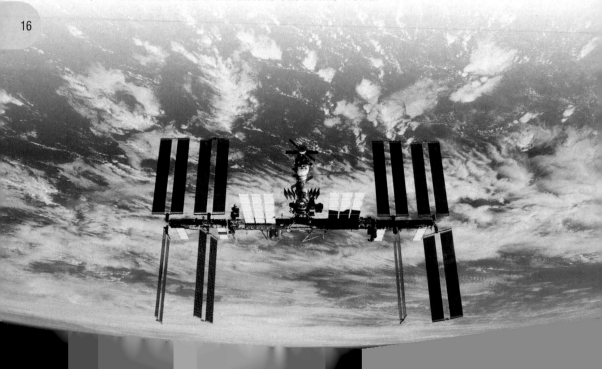

NUTRITION POWERHOUSE

Quinoa has earned its reputation as a superfood and a supergrain. When you look at how the nutrients in quinoa stack up compared to those in other grains, it's easy to understand why quinoa has garnered super status (see table 1, page 19). Quinoa is a whole grain, and it has twice the protein, fewer carbohydrates, and more healthy fats than other grains. It also has a great balance of essential amino acids (see table 2, page 21), which is why it's praised as a "complete protein," a rarity among plant-based foods.

Extraordinarily rich in certain minerals (including calcium, iron, magnesium, phosphorus, and potassium) and vitamins (including folate and vitamin E), quinoa also boasts exceptional amounts of dietary fiber. In addition, the grain is an excellent source of antioxidants. And finally, quinoa has a low glycemic index (see table 3, page 25), which means that it helps to regulate blood sugar levels.

According to research published in the *Journal of the Science of Food and Agriculture,* the minerals, vitamins, fatty acids, and antioxidants in quinoa strongly contribute to human nutrition. Beyond reducing the risks of various diseases, it's a food that is especially valuable in protecting cell membranes and supporting brain functions.

Whole Grain

Quinoa is considered a whole grain even though it's technically a seed and not a true grain, and the US Department of Agriculture (USDA) and many other sources include it on their lists of recommended whole grains. The USDA advises that we choose whole grains for at least half of the grains that we eat. In addition to quinoa, examples of whole grains include brown rice, buckwheat groats, bulgur (cracked wheat), millet, and whole-grain bread. If we follow the USDA's advice and make half of our grain intake whole grains, what would make up the other half? That would be refined grains, such as couscous, pearl barley, white bread, or white rice.

Quinoa provides all the health benefits attributed to whole grains, including reduced risk of cardiovascular disease (such as heart attack and stroke), type 2 diabetes, and certain kinds of cancer. In general, studies have shown that eating three daily servings of whole grains reduces the risk of cardiovascular disease and type 2 diabetes about equally, by between 20 and 30 percent. What's more, whole grains contribute significantly to digestive health by encouraging regularity, so there is less chance of constipation. Whole grains also protect against cancer,

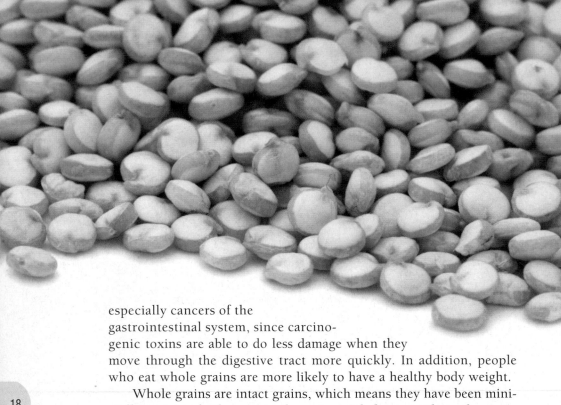

especially cancers of the
gastrointestinal system, since carcino-
genic toxins are able to do less damage when they
move through the digestive tract more quickly. In addition, people
who eat whole grains are more likely to have a healthy body weight.

    Whole grains are intact grains, which means they have been mini-
mally processed. They retain three essential elements: the endosperm,
the germ, and the bran. The endosperm is the large, starchy part of the
grain; the germ is the core that contains most of the fat, minerals, protein, and vitamins; and the bran is the outer layer, which contains most
of the fiber. As a pseudograin, quinoa's anatomy differs from the basic
three-part structure of cereal grains. Specifically, quinoa has a tail-like
germ that curls around the endosperm.

Quinoa in Comparison

Cooking with whole grains in general and quinoa in particular can rev up
nutrition in the kitchen. Quinoa is often recommended as a substitute for
rice, but it can be used in place of almost any other grain. It's easy and
convenient to cook and gives variety to menus. Quinoa also contributes a
unique texture and flavor, along with an outstanding nutritional profile.
Table 1 highlights the nutrient advantages quinoa has over other whole
grains and refined grains.

Nutrient Details

Take a look at table 1, and you'll quickly see that quinoa excels as a
source of select nutrients compared with other grains. There are a few

TABLE 1.

Nutrient comparison of one cup of cooked quinoa to one cup of other cooked grains

	BARLEY, PEARL	BUCKWHEAT GROATS, ROASTED	BULGUR	COUSCOUS	MILLET	QUINOA	RICE, LONG-GRAIN BROWN	RICE, LONG-GRAIN WHITE
Calories	193	155	151	176	207	**222**	216	205
Nutrient (in grams)								
Protein	3.55	5.68	5.61	5.95	6.11	**8.14**	5.03	4.25
Carbo-hydrates	44.31	33.5	33.82	36.46	41.19	**39.40**	44.77	44.51
Fat	.69	1.04	.44	.25	1.74	**3.55**	1.76	.44
Fiber	6.0	4.5	8.2	2.2	2.3	**5.2**	3.5	.60
Minerals (in milligrams)								
Calcium	17	12	18	13	5	**31**	20	16
Iron	2.09	1.34	1.75	.60	1.10	**2.76**	.82	1.9
Magnesium	35	86	58	13	77	**118**	84	19
Phosphorus	85	118	73	35	174	**281**	162	68
Potassium	146	148	124	91	108	**318**	84	55
Sodium	5	7	9	8	3	**13**	10	2
Zinc	1.29	1.02	1.04	.41	1.58	**2.02**	1.23	.77
Vitamins (in micrograms)								
Folate	25	24	33	24	33	**78**	8	153
Vitamin E	.02	.15	.02	.20	.03	**1.17**	.06	.06

Source: USDA National Nutrient Database for Standard Reference (http://ndb.nal.usda.gov)

exceptions. For example, pearl barley has slightly more fiber. In addition, several other grains have more carbohydrates, but that's not necessarily an advantage, especially when you consider the ratio of protein to carbohydrates (see Carbohydrates, page 20).

To give you a sense of how one cup of quinoa might satisfy your daily nutrient needs, estimated and recommended dietary allowances and average intakes are provided for each nutrient in the following sections. The recommendations for all nutrients were established by the Institute of Medicine.

Protein and Amino Acids

When it comes to nutrition, everyone seems to know about the importance of protein. It's necessary for building and repairing bones, muscles, and skin. But the foods most famous for their protein content, such as meat, eggs, and dairy products, can come with a walloping side of dangerous fats. That's not the case with quinoa and other grains, but most people don't give grains the credit they deserve when it comes to supplying this important nutrient. In fact, about half the protein in our diets comes from grains. And since quinoa can have up to 50 percent more protein than other grains, it's an overachiever in this category. One cup of cooked quinoa has more than 8 grams of protein. For adult males, the recommended protein intake is 56 grams per day; for adult females, it's 46 grams.

The proteins that we eat provide the amino acids in our diets. Quinoa is not only high in protein (14 to 20 percent protein), but it's also a high-quality protein because it has an exceptionally well-balanced amino acid profile, containing rich quantities of essential amino acids. The reason that certain amino acids are called "essential" is because our bodies can't create them on their own; we must get them through the foods we eat. And quinoa is one of the few plant-based foods that is considered a "complete protein" because of its protein quality. Table 2 (opposite page) lists the amounts of the essential amino acids in quinoa and other grains.

Quinoa has particularly high amounts of certain essential amino acids, including lysine and methionine. In fact, quinoa has about twice the amount of lysine as true cereal grains. Lysine is essential for muscle growth and repair, so it's important if you're interested in building muscle. In addition, lysine aids in the absorption of calcium and is involved in the production of antibodies, enzymes, and hormones.

Histidine, an amino acid that is essential for the growth of infants and children, is abundant in quinoa. The grain has been used traditionally as a weaning food in the Andes for many generations, and it's still an ideal early food for infants. Because it's easy to digest, quinoa can be given safely when introducing solid foods; well-cooked quinoa can be given to infants starting at age eight to ten months. Because the food is beneficial to young eaters, some authors have included recipes for quinoa-based foods for babies and children in quinoa cookbooks.

Carbohydrates

Whole grains, quinoa among them, are excellent sources of carbohydrates, and up to 85 percent of the calories in grains come from carbohydrates. This means whole grains are an outstanding source of energy. Quinoa is

TABLE 2. Amounts of essential amino acids in quinoa and other grains

ESSENTIAL AMINO ACIDS (in grams)	BARLEY, PEARL	BUCKWHEAT GROATS, ROASTED	BULGUR	COUSCOUS	MILLET	QUINOA	RICE, LONG-GRAIN BROWN	RICE, LONG-GRAIN WHITE
Histidine	.080	.133	.129	.121	.130	**.235**	.129	.100
Isoleucine	.130	.213	.207	.231	.258	**.290**	.213	.183
Leucine	.242	.356	.379	.407	.776	**.483**	.417	.351
Lysine	.132	.289	.155	.115	.117	**.442**	.193	.153
Methionine	.068	.074	.087	.093	.122	**.178**	.113	.100
Phenyla-lanine	.199	.223	.264	.289	.322	**.342**	.259	.228
Threonine	.121	.217	.162	.157	.197	**.242**	.185	.152
Tryptophan	.060	.082	.087	.077	.066	**.096**	.064	.049
Valine	.174	.291	.253	.254	.320	**.342**	.294	.259

Sources: USDA National Nutrient Database for Standard Reference (http://ndb.nal.usda.gov), US National Library of Medicine (for list of essential amino acids)

an exceptional power source any day, but it can be especially helpful when an extra boost is needed. For example, befitting its origin in the Andes, the grain is a favorite among mountain climbers because it gives them high endurance.

It's also worth noting that quinoa has a high ratio of protein to carbohydrates. Table 1 (page 19) shows that compared to other grains, quinoa has more protein and less carbohydrates. This means that people who eat quinoa feel full, or satiated, longer, which can be helpful in maintaining a healthy weight. The *British Journal of Nutrition* reported that when research subjects ate quinoa, they felt fuller than after eating rice or wheat.

One cup of cooked quinoa has nearly 40 grams of carbohydrates. For adults, the recommended carbohydrate intake is 130 grams per day.

Fat

The story about quinoa and fat is brief. Grains are naturally low in fat, and one cup of quinoa has less than 4 grams of fat. Quinoa contains no saturated fat, and like all plant-based foods, it has zero cholesterol. In comparison to most grains, quinoa has slightly more fat, but this only enhances its nutritional profile, since it has higher amounts of heart-healthy unsaturated fat than most grains.

Fiber

Grains that contain 5 to 7 grams of fiber per cup are considered high-fiber foods, and quinoa ranks in this category. Consuming adequate amounts of dietary fiber has a number of advantages. For one, it makes us feel good by keeping the contents of the gastrointestinal tract moving; in addition, it helps us feel satisfied after a meal. So fiber can potentially help us look good too, because high-fiber diets are associated with healthy body weights.

Fiber also plays an important role in controlling the levels of cholesterol and sugar in the blood, which reduces the risk of both cardiovascular disease and type 2 diabetes. As reported in the *Journal of the American Medical Association*, a lack of fiber in the diet directly correlates with the risk of heart attack, making fiber an important dietary component for the prevention of cardiovascular disease, particularly among men and older adults.

Adequate fiber intake is dictated considerably by gender and age. For adult males, the recommended total fiber intake is about 38 grams per day; those over age seventy require slightly less, about 30 grams. For adult females, the recommended total fiber intake is about 25 grams per day; those over age seventy require about 21 grams.

Minerals

Calcium

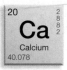

Everyone knows that calcium is needed for strong teeth and bones, but it has many other vital functions throughout the body, affecting muscle and blood vessel function, hormones and enzymes, nerve impulses, and more. While dairy foods are considered the heavyweights when it comes to providing calcium in the diet, there are many other contenders, including green vegetables, fruits, legumes, nuts, seeds, and nondairy milks. Grains aren't generally praised for supplying high amounts of calcium, but as a greater source of calcium than other grains, quinoa deserves an honorable mention, with about 31 milligrams per cup. The estimated average calcium requirement for adults is about 800 milligrams per day.

Iron

Among other tasks, the body needs iron to deliver oxygen to the blood. Once again, quinoa is a standout when compared with true cereal grains because it has four to six times more iron than these other grains. The 2.76 milligrams of iron per cup of quinoa goes a long way toward meeting estimated average requirements, which are 6 milligrams per day for adult males, 8 milligrams per day for adult women under age fifty, and 6 grams per day for women fifty and older.

Magnesium

One cup of quinoa has 118 milligrams of magnesium, which is critical for strong bones and cardiovascular health. Because it helps to relax blood vessels, magnesium can be helpful to people who have high blood pressure or migraine headaches. Quinoa is no slacker when it comes to magnesium content, given that the estimated average requirements are 350 milligrams for adult males and 265 milligrams for adult females.

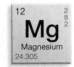

Phosphorus

Essential for forming bones and teeth, phosphorus also affects how the body uses carbohydrates and fats, among other important functions. With 281 milligrams of phosphorus per cup, quinoa is a mighty contributor to the estimated average requirement for adults, which is 580 milligrams per day.

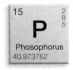

Potassium

As an essential mineral and an electrolyte, potassium affects every cell in our bodies. It helps nerves communicate with muscles, and in fact is responsible for every beat of our hearts. Many people are aware of the value of potassium and try to incorporate it into their diets to help control blood pressure and reduce the risk of cardiovascular disease. Vegetables and fruits are rightfully credited with supplying rich amounts of potassium, but whole grains are also valuable sources. None rivals quinoa, however, which ranks highest among all grains in potassium content. One cup of quinoa has .318 grams of potassium, and the adequate intake for adults is 4.7 grams per day.

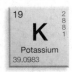

Sodium

Our bodies, especially the nerves and muscles, need sodium to function properly. However, most people are worried about getting too much sodium in their diets, which can lead to high blood pressure and other health problems. Even though quinoa has more sodium than other grains, the amount it contains is still very low. One cup has only .013 gram, and the recommended intake for adults is 1.5 grams.

Vitamins

Folate and B Vitamins

Quinoa is high in folate and other B vitamins, which help prevent cardio-vascular, nerve, and skin disorders. In particular, folate is essential in the formation of red blood cells, creating and repairing DNA, and cell division and growth. Folate can reduce the risk of birth defects, and women who may become pregnant are advised to consume adequate amounts of folate to avoid neurological birth defects. For pregnant women, estimated requirements are 530 micrograms of folate per day. For other adults, the requirement is 320 micrograms. One cup of quinoa contains 78 micrograms of folate.

Vitamin E

As a powerful antioxidant, vitamin E provides overall protection from disease. Oils, nuts, and seeds are rich sources of vitamin E, and since quinoa is technically a seed rather than a grain, it's no surprise that it has more vitamin E than grains. One cup of quinoa has 1.78 micrograms of vitamin E, and the average requirement for adults is 12 micrograms.

Other Nutritional Benefits

Antioxidants

Also known as phytochemicals, antioxidants are, quite simply, chemi-cals that originate from a plant. When we eat plant-based foods, these antioxidants give us abundant health advantages. They protect against many kinds of illness, combat degenerative disease, and potentially con-tribute to overall lifespan. Antioxidants are divided into different types, including flavonoids. Research reported in the journal *Food Chemistry* has shown that the flavonoid content of quinoa is exceptionally high. The two flavonoids found in quinoa are kaempferol and quercetin. Sur-prisingly, researchers stated that quinoa's concentrated content of these powerful antioxidants is superior to that of berries, such as cranberries, which have long ranked as high-flavonoid food sources.

A separate study reported in the *Journal of Medicinal Food* dem-onstrated that quinoa may be helpful in managing type 2 diabetes and associated hypertension because it's especially rich in quercetin and other antioxidants. Among the ten traditional Peruvian grains and legumes studied, quinoa had the highest overall antioxidant activity (86 percent).

Glycemic Index

In addition to all of its other virtues, quinoa is a food with a low glyce-mic index (GI). This index ranks carbohydrates according to how they

TABLE 3. Glycemic index (GI) of cooked quinoa compared to other cooked grains

	BARLEY, PEARL	BUCKWHEAT GROATS, ROASTED	BULGUR	COUSCOUS	MILLET	QUINOA	RICE, LONG-GRAIN BROWN	RICE, LONG-GRAIN WHITE
Glycemic index	35	51	46	65	71	**53**	72	76

Source: University of Sydney (glycemicindex.com)

Key: Glycemic values follow: low-GI foods have a value of 55 or less; medium-GI foods have a value of 56 to 69; and high-GI foods have a value of 70 or more.

affect blood glucose levels. Foods with a low GI value are digested slowly, releasing glucose gradually into the bloodstream, helping to reduce blood glucose levels throughout the day and keeping you off the blood-sugar roller coaster. These types of foods are helpful in preventing heart disease and type 2 diabetes. They also can help you lose weight because they make you feel full and keep you satisfied longer; in addition, they help burn more body fat.

Table 3 (above) lists the GI values of quinoa and other cooked grains. Whole grains, like quinoa, tend to have a low GI, whereas refined grains, such as white rice, typically have higher GI values. Low-GI foods cause gentle rises in blood glucose levels compared to high-GI foods, which cause levels to spike. When blood sugar is high, the body releases greater amounts of insulin to manage it, either by using it as energy, storing it as a form of glucose, or converting it into fat. That's why eating foods with a low GI value is important in controlling the body's insulin levels, which is critical in preventing and managing diabetes. As reported in the *American Journal of Clinical Nutrition*, eating a low-GI diet can be as important in preventing heart disease and type 2 diabetes as eating a whole-grain, high-fiber diet.

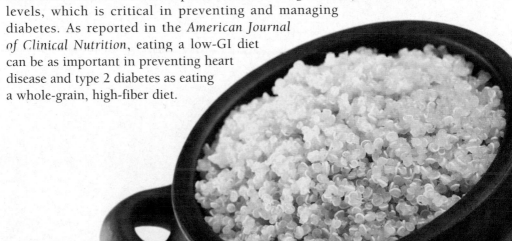

QUINOA, THE GLUTEN-FREE GRAIN

A ccording to the Food and Agriculture Organization of the United Nations, quinoa is the only gluten-free crop that has all of the essential amino acids, trace elements, and vitamins needed by the human body. The previous section (Nutrition Powerhouse, page 17) reviewed all of the wonderful nutrients that quinoa contains, but this statement is an important reminder that for some people, quinoa's value lies not only in what it does contain but also in what it doesn't, and that's gluten.

What is gluten? Gluten is a protein found in wheat, barley, and rye. Hard to avoid in North American cuisine, gluten lurks in many mainstream foods, from baked goods to pasta to sandwiches, mainly in the form of wheat flour (including all-purpose flour and whole wheat flour). The main ingredient in most breads, gluten-containing wheat flour gives bread elasticity and cohesiveness. In fact, the term comes from the Latin word *gluten*, which means "glue." But bread and other products made from wheat flour aren't the only sources of gluten; many processed foods and products, including some you wouldn't expect, also contain gluten (see sidebar, opposite page).

For most people, eating gluten isn't a problem. For others, such as those with celiac disease or gluten sensitivity, gluten brings debilitating symptoms and the risk for serious health complications. One excellent strategy for replacing gluten in the diet is to include quinoa in all its forms—the grain, flakes, flour, and pasta. Quinoa doesn't contain gluten because it's not a member of the same plant family as wheat, which is a cereal grass. This makes quinoa a nutritious and recommended option for people who have celiac disease or gluten sensitivity.

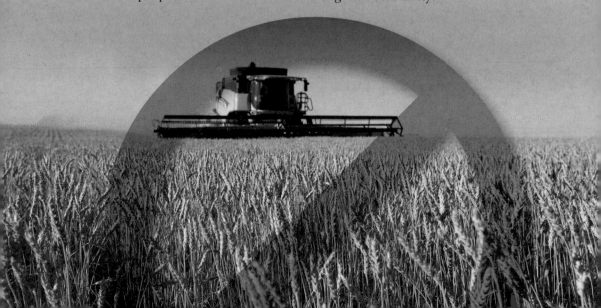

FOODS AND PRODUCTS THAT CONTAIN GLUTEN

In addition to avoiding obvious gluten-containing foods—such as barley, bulgur, rye, wheat, and wheat pasta and flours—there are a number of processed foods and other products that may be unexpected sources of gluten. While some of the following items are available gluten-free, always read labels and err on the side of caution:

- beer
- bouillon cubes
- brown rice syrup
- candy
- communion wafers
- French fries
- herbal and nutritional supplements
- lip balm
- malt
- matzo
- medicine
- salad dressing
- sauces and gravies
- seasoned chips and snack foods
- soups and soup bases
- soy sauce
- vitamins and mineral supplements

Celiac Disease and Gluten Sensitivity

Celiac disease, which is sometimes called celiac sprue, is an autoimmune condition affecting both children and adults. When people with celiac disease eat gluten, it causes a toxic reaction that damages the small intestine and prevents food from being properly absorbed. Minute amounts of gluten can cause health problems and damage to the small intestine, even when the person afflicted may appear to have no symptoms.

People who have celiac disease must scrupulously avoid all gluten-containing foods. Gluten protein is found in all forms of wheat, including durum, semolina, spelt, Kamut, einkorn, and faro. It's also found in botanically related grains, including rye, barley, and triticale. No foods made with these grains or that have come in contact with them can be consumed by someone who has celiac disease.

People who have a gluten sensitivity or intolerance but who don't have celiac disease don't experience damage to the small intestine from gluten. Although their sensitivity may not be life-threatening, their symptoms (typically gastrointestinal) are often debilitating. Therefore, they also need to avoid all foods that contain gluten.

Fortunately, the various forms of quinoa—ranging from the whole grain to pasta to flakes to flour—are almost always gluten-free and safe for those with celiac disease. Nevertheless, always read package labels to be certain (and never purchase quinoa products from the bulk bin,

QUINOA AND OTHER SAFE GRAINS AND SEEDS

People who have celiac disease or gluten sensitivity can include the following grains and seeds in their diets:

- amaranth
- arrowroot
- buckwheat
- corn
- flax
- legumes
- millet
- oats (see page 32)
- quinoa
- rice
- seeds (such as pumpkin, sesame, and sunflower)
- sorghum
- teff
- wild rice

as they may be cross-contaminated with gluten-containing foods). For a list of safe grains and seeds, see the sidebar above.

People with celiac disease face symptoms that are wide and varied, and the disease affects individuals differently. They can have a number of digestive symptoms, such as abdominal bloating, pain, chronic diarrhea, and constipation. They can also experience symptoms that affect other parts of the body, such as anemia, arthritis, depression, osteoporosis, a skin rash called dermatitis herpetiformis, and sores in the mouth.

According to a study by the Center for Celiac Research and Treatment in Boston, more than two million, or about 1 in 133, people in the United States have the disease, and many adults have it for a decade or longer before they're diagnosed. Because the symptoms experienced by people with celiac disease are often attributed to other health problems, such as irritable bowel syndrome or Crohn's disease, it can be difficult to get a definitive diagnosis, which is done through blood tests and a biopsy of the small intestine. If you suspect you have celiac disease but haven't been tested, it's important to maintain a typical diet; that is, don't go gluten-free until after undergoing medical testing or you may get false negative results.

An estimated eighteen million people, or 6 percent of the US population, have gluten sensitivity but don't have celiac disease. The symptoms of gluten sensitivity are similar to those of celiac disease; however, unlike celiac disease, gluten sensitivity doesn't result in intestinal inflammation or damage to the small intestine. As a result, people with gluten sensitivity don't face the same long-term damage to the small intestine as those with celiac disease.

The only way to treat celiac disease or gluten sensitivity is to eliminate all gluten from the diet, which allows the small intestine to heal and the proper absorption of nutrients to resume. Until other treatments are available, this means that people with celiac disease must practice a gluten-free diet consistently, or they risk escalation of the disease in addition to the development of related complications. Untreated celiac disease can be life threatening. Long-term malabsorption of nutrients can lead to nervous system disorders, osteoporosis, and disease of the gallbladder, liver, pancreas, and spleen. Untreated celiac disease is also associated with risk for specific types of cancer, including intestinal lymphoma.

The good news is that within days of eliminating gluten from the diet, people with celiac disease and gluten sensitivity can expect to see improvement in their symptoms and experience some relief. And there's more good news: Awareness about the needs of those who live gluten-free is growing. Food manufacturers and restaurant managers are becoming increasingly mindful of consumers' needs and are making more appropriate options available. In addition, many authors have written on the topic, and numerous gluten-free cookbooks are now on the market. Several organizations provide support and information online (see Resources, page 60), making it easier than ever to switch to a gluten-free diet. One excellent strategy is to replace gluten-containing foods with quinoa products, including the grain, flakes, flour, and pasta.

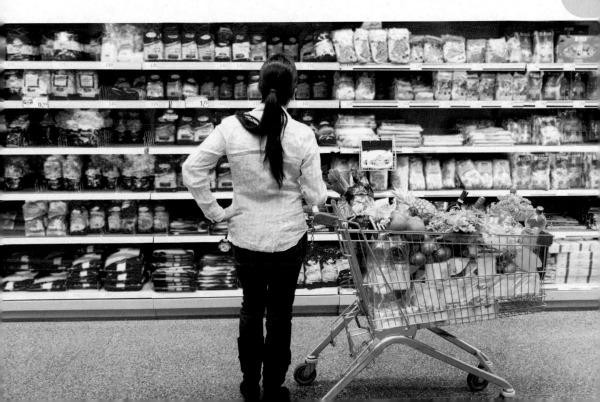

Quinoa in the Gluten-Free Diet

Simple adjustments can make quinoa a star player in your gluten-free routine. For example, using the grain as a side dish or in grain salads is easy to do. And replacing standard wheat-based pasta with quinoa pasta is a no-brainer. Table 4 (below) provides a list of convenient ways to replace gluten-containing products with quinoa.

If you're adept at baking, living gluten-free doesn't mean living without baked goods. Quinoa flour and other gluten-free flours can be substituted for all-purpose wheat flour in many recipes. As described in the following section (Cooking with Quinoa, page 33), quinoa flour can be used exclusively, or it can be mixed with other gluten-free flours, such as arrowroot or buckwheat, to achieve the desired texture and flavor. Another option is to seek out gluten-free baking mixes in natural food stores or online. While some of these products may include small amounts of quinoa flour, they're more likely to contain less nutritious alternatives. Many of the mixes use rice flour as a key ingredient. Such baking mixes can be costly and lack nutrition, so experimenting on your own with wholesome quinoa flour can be a wise alternative. Incorporating quinoa flour into baked goods gives them a big nutritional boost. In fact, according to the journal *Food Chemistry*, gluten-free products made with quinoa have significantly greater amounts of polyphenols and antioxidants than gluten-free products made from corn, potato, or rice.

TABLE 4. Quinoa substitutions for gluten-containing foods

FOODS WITH GLUTEN	QUINOA ALTERNATIVE
Bulgur, cooked (in tabouli or other grain salads)	Quinoa grain, cooked
Breadcrumbs (to coat other foods; to top casseroles)	Quinoa flakes
Couscous, cooked (as a side dish or in stews)	Quinoa grain, cooked
Oatmeal (in granola, muesli, porridge, cookies, and muffins)	Quinoa flakes
Thickener for smoothies or soups	Quinoa flakes
Wheat flour (including all-purpose flour)	Quinoa flour or a combination of quinoa flour and another gluten-free flour
Wheat pasta	Quinoa pasta

BEWARE THE BULK SECTION

If your health requires that you avoid gluten, it's safe to eat quinoa. However, it may not be safe to eat quinoa (or any other food) that's sold in bulk bins at natural food stores or supermarkets. There are countless ways that bulk foods can be cross-contaminated with gluten, making even naturally gluten-free foods risky to consume if they were purchased in the bulk section. For those who are sensitive to gluten and must avoid health risks, the prudent choice is to purchase quinoa products in packages that indicate the contents were processed in a gluten-free facility.

Additional research has shown the benefits of incorporating quinoa into a gluten-free diet, especially in terms of adding vital nutrients, such as protein, and decreasing fat intake. The *Journal of Human Nutrition and Dietetics* noted that adding quinoa instead of rice, a standard gluten-free option, to meals and snacks increased nutrition, especially levels of protein (20.6 grams versus 11 grams), iron (18.4 milligrams versus 1.4 milligrams), calcium (182 milligrams versus 0 milligrams), and fiber (12.7 grams versus 5 grams). The *European Journal of Nutrition* reported that research subjects were evaluated for blood lipid levels (free fatty acid levels and triglyceride concentrations) after eating gluten-free foods. Study participants had lower lipid levels after eating quinoa than after eating gluten-free pastas and breads, making quinoa a standout in this study.

An article published in the journal *Nutrients* discussed the role of quinoa and other gluten-free grains in gluten-free diets, which are frequently poor in nutritional content. Studies have shown that 20 to 38 percent of people with celiac disease are deficient in common nutrients, including dietary fiber, minerals, and vitamins. Inadequate fiber intake likely occurs because many gluten-free foods are made with starches or refined flour with low fiber content. Furthermore, gluten-free diets often are high in calories, animal protein, and fat, which can contribute to weight gain and increase health risks, such as coronary heart disease. The authors of the article recommended quinoa as one gluten-free grain that could improve overall nutrition by increasing fiber intake, vitamin (especially folate) intake, and mineral intake. In fact, the authors emphasized that the total content of minerals in amaranth, quinoa, and oats is about twice as high as that in other cereals. In addition, quinoa's antioxidant content can be of benefit to those on a gluten-free diet; research has shown that buckwheat and quinoa have the highest antioxidant potential among studied cereals and pseudocereals.

While health authorities have consistently recommended quinoa as a safe gluten-free food, new research suggests that a modest percentage of quinoa strains may contain small amounts of gluten. One study reported in the *American Journal of Clinical Nutrition* examined fifteen varieties of quinoa from Peru. Of these, four strains had measurable concentrations of celiac-toxic epitopes, which are substances that can elicit an immune response. These levels, however, fall below the maximum permitted for gluten-free food. Researchers concluded that while most quinoa cultivars have no quantifiable concentrations of celiac-toxic epitopes, some cultivars could cause an immune response in people with celiac disease. Since quinoa is such an important source of nutrients for those who can't tolerate gluten, researchers recommend further investigation. In the meantime, those who eat gluten-free can observe their response to quinoa and adjust their diets accordingly.

Specific Concerns about Oats

People who have celiac disease or gluten sensitivity have routinely been warned about eating oats. At one time, scientists were concerned about the proteins in oats, suspecting that they caused effects similar to gluten, which is the primary protein in wheat. New evidence, however, shows that the body's response to gluten is significantly different than its response to the protein in oats. As a result, people with celiac disease are typically advised that it's safe to eat oats in moderation if they can tolerate them. The responsibility lies with the consumer here, because it's essential to eat only oats that aren't contaminated with wheat gluten, which sometimes occurs during processing and transport.

If you want to try oats, check labels or call the manufacturer to confirm whether a specific brand of oats is free of gluten contamination. Or, if you prefer, another option is to substitute quinoa flakes in any recipe that calls for oats. From the standard breakfast porridge to baked goods, quinoa flakes are an excellent stand-in for oats.

Dairy Products May Also Be a Concern

People who have celiac disease may also be sensitive to the proteins and sugar (lactose) in cow's milk. In fact, half of all people with celiac disease are also lactose intolerant.

If you've been diagnosed with celiac disease and have found that a gluten-free diet doesn't eliminate your symptoms, avoiding dairy products may be the solution you're looking for. Many alternatives to cow's milk are sold commercially or can be made at home. Almond, rice, and soy milk are readily available. Although there's currently no commercial form of quinoa milk, several enterprising cooks have provided online instructions on how to whip up a batch at home.

COOKING WITH QUINOA

Quinoa is a culinary delight. Endlessly versatile, it can be substituted for almost any other grain in all kinds of recipes, and it works equally well in savory or sweet dishes. Here's your guide to the types of quinoa products that are available, where to find them, and how to use them. Also included are pointers for cooking or sprouting the grain.

Forms of Quinoa

One reason that quinoa is such a versatile ingredient is because it comes in a variety of colors and forms, including the grain itself, flakes, flour, and pasta. Look for these products in natural food stores and most supermarkets. You may get the best deal if you can find these items in the bulk section. Although this can be an affordable option, it can also be a potentially dangerous one if you must eat gluten-free. Foods that are stored in bulk containers that allow consumers to help themselves, or that are interchanged with other bulk containers, are easily cross-contaminated (see sidebar, page 31).

Although they're increasingly available in natural food stores and even some supermarkets, red and black quinoa and quinoa flakes may be a little more difficult to find than white quinoa, quinoa flour, and quinoa pasta. If you can't find these products locally, there are many good online sources (see Resources, page 60).

The Grain

Although quinoa can come in a range of colors, the three commercially available varieties are white, red, and black. In general, the lighter the color, the milder the flavor, and the darker the color, the chewier or crunchier the texture. The colored varieties can be substituted in any recipe that calls for white quinoa. To make any quinoa dish visually and texturally interesting, combine different colors of quinoa. This simple step can be made even easier if you're lucky enough to find a package of "rainbow quinoa," which already contains white, red, and black quinoa.

No matter which color of quinoa you choose, the cooking method (see pages 37–39) is the same. Red and black quinoa, however, may take slightly longer to cook than white quinoa. Both red and black quinoa retain their dramatic color when cooked.

Like other whole grains, store quinoa of all colors in a cool, dark, and dry place. Because quinoa is a seed with a fairly high oil content, it's a good idea to store uncooked quinoa in the refrigerator, preferably in tightly sealed containers or glass jars.

WHITE QUINOA. The most common and affordable type of quinoa, white quinoa is usually just labeled "quinoa" and appears cream, ivory, or pale yellow in color. Mild, mellow, and slightly nutty, white quinoa can be substituted in recipes for just about any grain and will complement all kinds of ingredients that pair naturally with grains, including legumes and vegetables.

RED QUINOA. Like tiny mahogany beads, red quinoa grains are a deep reddish brown. Red quinoa is firmer when cooked than white quinoa and holds its shape well, which makes it an excellent choice for grain salads or other recipes in which the grain should remain distinct. Red quinoa also is chewier than white quinoa, and its flavor is nuttier.

BLACK QUINOA. Black or very dark brown, black quinoa may be a bit firmer and crunchier after cooking than the white or red varieties. It also has a stronger flavor, which has been described as earthy and sweet.

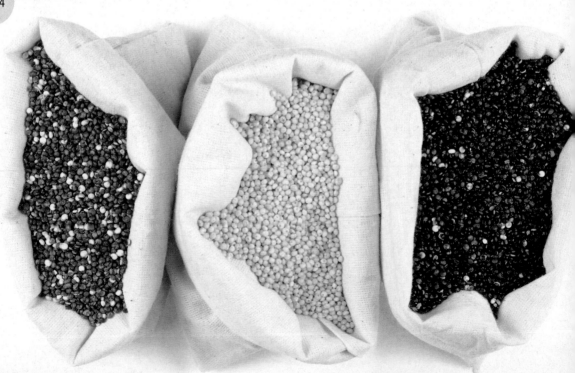

EASY WAYS TO USE QUINOA

Whether you're dishing up breakfast, lunch, dinner, or dessert, quinoa in its many forms provides plentiful nutritious options.

COOKED QUINOA

- add to a hearty stew or chili
- serve as a plain side dish
- combine with other grains in a pilaf
- make a stuffing for bell peppers, mushrooms, or squash
- mix with black beans, corn, and salsa for a classic salad
- stir into bean dip or hummus for a nutrient boost
- substitute for arborio rice in risotto or for bulgur in tabouli
- use instead of rice to make a sweet, creamy pudding

SPROUTED QUINOA

- add to cereals or other cold dishes
- top a salad of fresh greens
- use as a sandwich filling
- garnish a gourmet dish

QUINOA FLAKES

- blend into a smoothie for added protein
- make a quick and easy breakfast porridge
- substitute for breadcrumbs to coat foods before cooking
- thicken soups and stews
- use like rolled oats when baking cookies or muffins

QUINOA FLOUR

- bake gluten-free cookies and other goodies
- make pancake and waffle batter
- use alone or in combination with other flours

Quinoa Flakes

Like rolled oats, quinoa flakes are made by steamrolling the whole grain. In this case, whole white quinoa is steamrolled after the bitter saponin layer has been removed. Like quick oats, quinoa flakes cook in mere minutes, making an almost instant breakfast porridge that's similar to oatmeal. This nonallergenic and rather bland food is a good choice for babies who are beginning to eat solid foods; older children and adults may prefer quinoa porridge enhanced with fresh or dried fruits, nuts, sweeteners, or spices.

Quinoa flakes can double for oats in all kinds of recipes, including granola, muesli, cookies, and muffins. They also can be substituted for breadcrumbs when coating foods, mixed into a savory pilaf, used as binder in veggie burgers, stirred into soup as a thickener, or blended into a smoothie to add protein. For the best results, store quinoa flakes in a sealed container in the refrigerator or freezer.

Quinoa Flour

Ground from whole white quinoa seeds, quinoa flour increases the protein and nutrient-quality of baked goods. It's an excellent and versatile choice whether or not your goal is to bake gluten-free.

Quinoa flour is light and has a texture similar to all-purpose wheat flour. Typically pale yellow in color, quinoa flour is slightly darker than all-purpose flour, which can make baked goods a bit darker too. And because quinoa flour is gluten-free, it can also produce a denser texture than all-purpose flour. Some commercial brands are coarser than others; for the best results when baking, use finely ground quinoa flour. One option is to make your own quinoa flour at home (see sidebar, page 37).

Raw quinoa flour is sometimes described as having an "earthy" smell, which newcomers might find surprising and even unpleasant. However, baked goods made with quinoa flour have a distinctive nutty flavor, which many people find appealing. If the flavor seems particularly strong to you, one solution is to use quinoa flour in recipes that have other strong-tasting ingredients, such as cocoa, extracts, and spices. Pairing these robust flavors can be wonderfully complementary.

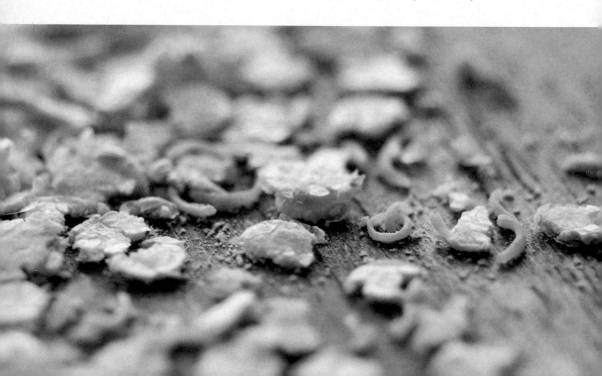

MAKE QUINOA FLOUR AT HOME

It's easy and affordable to make quinoa flour at home. Simply put uncooked white quinoa seeds into a coffee grinder or grain mill to produce a fine flour. About ¾ cup of quinoa seeds will make 1 cup of quinoa flour. By grinding quinoa flour at home as you need it, you'll be using the freshest, most nutritious ingredient possible.

If your goal is to create gluten-free products, you can use 100 percent quinoa flour to make cakes, cookies, pancakes, and waffles. For a milder flavor, consider combining quinoa flour with another gluten-free flour, such as amaranth or millet flour. If you're not baking gluten-free, you can use half all-purpose wheat flour and half quinoa flour in most recipes for baked goods. Keep in mind that batters made with quinoa flour won't rise like those made with all-purpose wheat flour, and some recipes may need additional leavening.

Because of the oils they contain, all whole-grain flours may become rancid over time. For the longest shelf life, store quinoa flour in a sealed container in the refrigerator for two to three months or in the freezer for six to eight months.

Quinoa Pasta

Gluten-free quinoa flour is made into several types of pasta by various manufacturers. It has an appealing texture and flavor that is quite similar to regular wheat-based pasta. Most manufacturers combine quinoa with another gluten-free grain ingredient, such as corn or rice flour. Check labels if you have any concerns about food allergies or sensitivities.

If you're new to quinoa pasta, follow the cooking directions on the package and test for doneness frequently to make sure the noodles aren't undercooked or getting overcooked. Then use the cooked pasta as you would any other type of pasta in your favorite recipes.

Best Quinoa Cooking Method

Here's the modern secret for cooking this ancient grain. This method is summarized in the Basic Quinoa recipe (page 42).

Note that this method departs significantly from those you'll see on most product labels and in many cookbooks. If you use this cooking method, your quinoa will turn out more dense and tender and won't retain the characteristic crunch that can make it seem undercooked. What's more, when it's cooked this way, quinoa doesn't turn into a mushy lump. Instead, the grain remains firm and distinct (like rice) and can be used in countless dishes, such as stirred into a robust salad. For best results when making grain salads, cook the quinoa first, and let it cool before combining it with other ingredients.

1. Soak the quinoa (optional). Soaking the quinoa for at least 5 minutes before cooking will help remove any bitterness or coatings and soften the grain. Soaking is optional but recommended, especially for quinoa purchased in bulk or from questionable producers (plus, it doesn't take very long).

2. Rinse the quinoa (optional, unless the quinoa hasn't been pre-rinsed). After a short optional soak, the quinoa should be drained in a fine-mesh strainer and rinsed well. As described on page 6, quinoa has a bitter coating, called the saponin layer, which acts as a natural deterrent to pests. Most quinoa that's sold today has been processed so that the saponin is removed, but it's still a good idea to rinse the quinoa thoroughly at home to remove any lingering remnants or bitterness. If you're fortunate enough to find a brand of quinoa that you trust has been thoroughly washed and states on the label that no rinsing is required, lucky you! In that case, you can skip this step if you prefer.

To rinse the quinoa, put it in a fine-mesh strainer; because the grains are so tiny, they'll fall through the holes of ordinary colanders. Rinse the quinoa under running water, rubbing the grains together gently between your fingers to remove any saponin. Don't be surprised if you see a soapy lather from the saponin—just keep rinsing until the water runs clear and no lather remains. If you can detect any bitterness in cooked quinoa and plan to cook grains from the same batch in the future, you may want to soak the quinoa for 1 to 2 hours before rinsing thoroughly.

3. Toast the quinoa (optional). Toasting the quinoa will improve the flavor, enhancing its naturally nutty taste, so this step is recommended (but not required). To toast, put the rinsed quinoa (it's okay if the quinoa is still damp) in a skillet or saucepan over medium-high heat. If desired, add 2 teaspoons of olive oil to further enhance the flavor. Toast the quinoa, stirring occasionally, until the grains are dry and fragrant, about 5 minutes. Remove the skillet or the saucepan from the heat. If you used a skillet to toast the quinoa, transfer the quinoa to a saucepan before adding the water and cooking. If you toasted the quinoa in a saucepan, you can add the water and cook the quinoa in the same saucepan. Stand back when adding the water as it might sputter.

4. Use less water. Most package instructions and cookbooks recommend using one part quinoa and two parts water when cooking. The method recommended in this book departs significantly from that old standard, which has done the great grain a disservice and may have turned off legions of potential fans because this ratio results in a cooked grain with an unappealing and mushy consistency. When it comes to cooking quinoa, using less water is the key to success. To make about 3 cups of cooked quinoa, put 1 cup of toasted quinoa and 1¼ cups of water in a saucepan. This will make 2 to 4 servings, depending on whether the quinoa will be served as a side dish or main dish and what other ingredients will be added to it.

5. Cook for a full 30 minutes. Bring to a boil over high heat. After it comes to a boil, decrease the heat to low, cover, and cook for a full 30 minutes (use a timer). Note, once again, that these instructions defy conventional recommendations, which generally advise cooking quinoa for only 10 to 20 minutes. This short cooking time, however, results in a grain with an unappealing and often crunchy texture.

There's no need to remove the cover from the saucepan or stir quinoa while it's cooking. In fact, stirring is discouraged because whole grains bruise easily, and stirring can make them sticky.

After the quinoa has cooked for the full 30 minutes, check it for doneness. It's easy to tell when quinoa is done cooking because the germ, which looks like a little white tail, pops out and curls around the grain, which should be translucent and plump. Sample the quinoa, especially to observe the texture. Do you prefer it with a bit of crunch or more tender? If you want a more tender grain, allow it to cook or sit in the covered saucepan just a bit longer, then test again. It's important not to overcook quinoa, which will turn to mush. Note that red or black quinoa tends to be crunchier and may need a slightly longer cooking time.

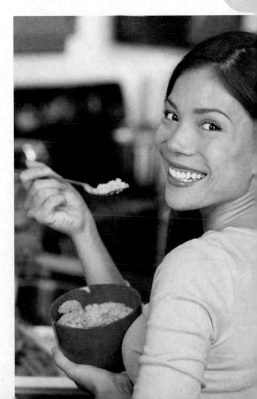

When the quinoa is done cooking, remove the saucepan from the heat and let sit, covered, for 5 minutes. Fluff with a fork before serving.

You may be surprised to see how much grain this recipe yields. Although the grains are tiny, quinoa expands about three times its original volume when cooked in water or broth. Stored in a sealed container, leftover cooked quinoa will keep in the refrigerator for 5 days. So consider making a large batch that can be used throughout the week in a variety of dishes.

Sprouting Quinoa

Quinoa can be sprouted and used in cereals, salads, sandwiches, and even cold main dishes. Before sprouting quinoa, rinse it thoroughly to remove the bitter saponin layer, just as you would before cooking the grain. Sprouting may even be more successful if the saponin wasn't mechanically removed by the distributor, since some quinoa might not sprout if the germ has been nipped during the saponin removal process. If you're not able to make regular quinoa sprout, try using seed-quality quinoa that retains its saponin layer (the seeds are available through seed catalogs and websites; see Resources, page 60). Just be sure to rinse the quinoa seeds very thoroughly before sprouting. Put the seeds in a fine-mesh strainer under running water until the water runs clear.

Quinoa is a very quick sprouter, growing about one inch after just two days. By the third day, the sprout is ready, displaying a beautiful red stem and bright green leaf.

To sprout quinoa, put $\frac{1}{3}$ cup of the seeds in a sprouting jar covered with a sprouting lid or cheesecloth secured with a rubber band. Add enough water to cover the seeds and let soak for 2 to 4 hours. Drain the water and let the jar stand upside down in the dish drainer. Rinse the seeds 2 to 3 times daily with fresh water, and drain by letting the jar stand upside down in the dish drainer after each rinsing.

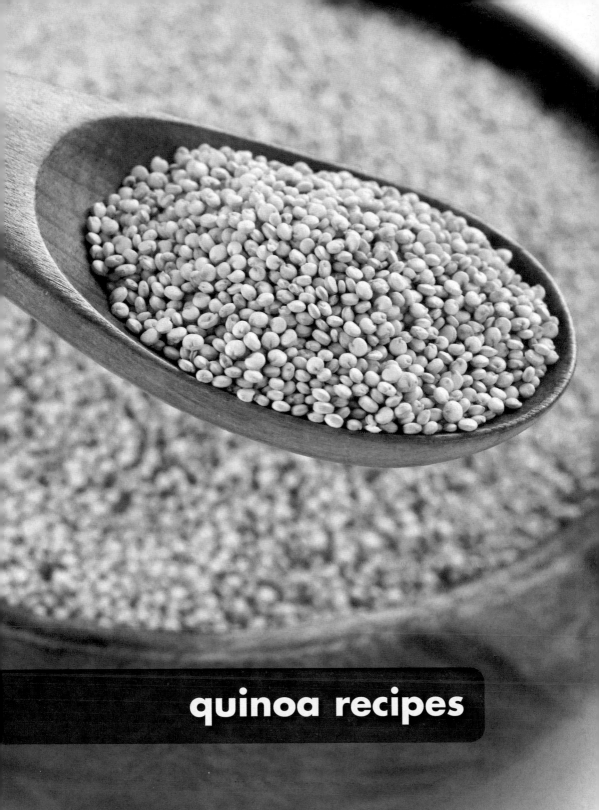

quinoa recipes

basic Quinoa

Use this indispensable recipe as the foundation for any dish that calls for cooked quinoa, such as pilafs, salads, side dishes, and desserts.

1 cup **quinoa**

2 teaspoons **olive oil** (optional)

1¼ cups **water**

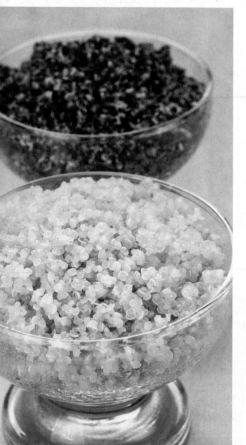

Put the quinoa in a fine-mesh strainer. If time permits, briefly soak the quinoa. To do this, put the strainer in a medium bowl and add enough water to cover the quinoa. Let soak for 5 minutes. Drain, rinse well under running water, stirring the quinoa with your fingers, and drain again. If time is short, simply rinse the quinoa well, stirring with your fingers, and drain.

If desired, toast the quinoa. Put the soaked or rinsed quinoa in a medium saucepan or skillet over medium-high heat. Add the optional oil (the oil will further enhance the flavor of the quinoa). Toast the quinoa, stirring occasionally, until the grains are dry and fragrant, about 5 minutes. Remove the skillet or the saucepan from the heat. If you used a skillet to toast the quinoa, transfer the quinoa to a medium saucepan before proceeding. If you toasted the quinoa in a saucepan, you can cook the quinoa in the same saucepan.

Add the water to the saucepan and bring to a boil over high heat. If you used oil to toast the quinoa, stand back when adding the water as it may sputter. Decrease the heat to low, cover, and cook for 30 minutes. Remove from the heat and let stand, covered, for 5 minutes. Fluff with a fork and serve at once, use in other recipes, or store in a covered container in the refrigerator for up to 5 days.

Quinoa-Oat *porridge*

This satisfying hot breakfast cereal gets the morning off right, with fiber, fruit, and flavor galore.

½ cup **water**

¼ cup **white quinoa, soaked, rinsed, and drained (see page 38)**

1 cup **vanilla nondairy milk**

½ cup **quick-cooking rolled oats**

¼ teaspoon **ground cinnamon**

¼ teaspoon **salt (optional)**

1 cup peeled and diced **apple**

1 tablespoon **maple syrup**

2 tablespoons **chopped walnuts**

Put the water in a medium saucepan and bring to a boil over high heat. Stir in the quinoa, decrease the heat to low, cover, and cook until most of the water is absorbed, about 20 minutes.

Add the nondairy milk, oats, cinnamon, and optional salt. Bring to a boil over high heat. Decrease the heat to medium-low and cook, stirring often, until thick and creamy, about 4 minutes. Stir in the apple and remove from the heat. Portion into two bowls and top with the maple syrup and walnuts.

43

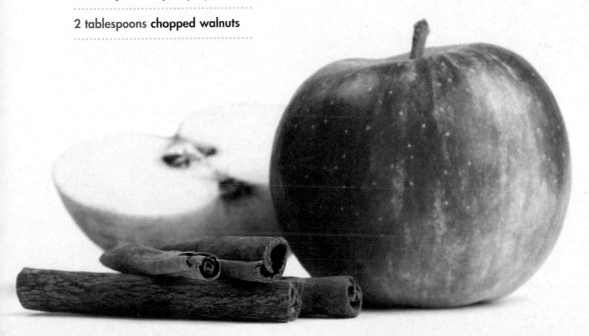

blueberry **Breakfast Quinoa**

This sweet porridge is packed with protein from the quinoa, antioxidants from the blueberries, and crunchy goodness from the sunflower seeds.

2 cups **vanilla nondairy milk**

1 cup **quinoa, soaked, rinsed, and drained (see page 38)**

Pinch **salt (optional)**

3 tablespoons **maple syrup**

1 teaspoon **lemon zest**

1 cup **blueberries**

2 tablespoons **unsalted toasted sunflower seeds**

Heat the nondairy milk in a medium saucepan over medium heat until warm, 2 to 3 minutes. Stir in the quinoa and optional salt. Decrease the heat to medium-low, cover, and cook until most of the liquid has been absorbed, about 30 minutes. Remove from the heat. Stir in the maple syrup and lemon zest. Gently fold in the blueberries.

Portion into two bowls. Top each serving with 1 tablespoon of the sunflower seeds.

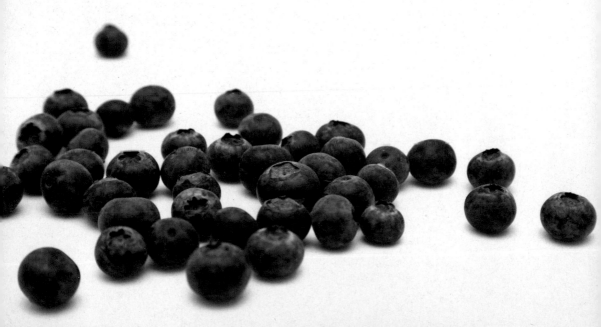

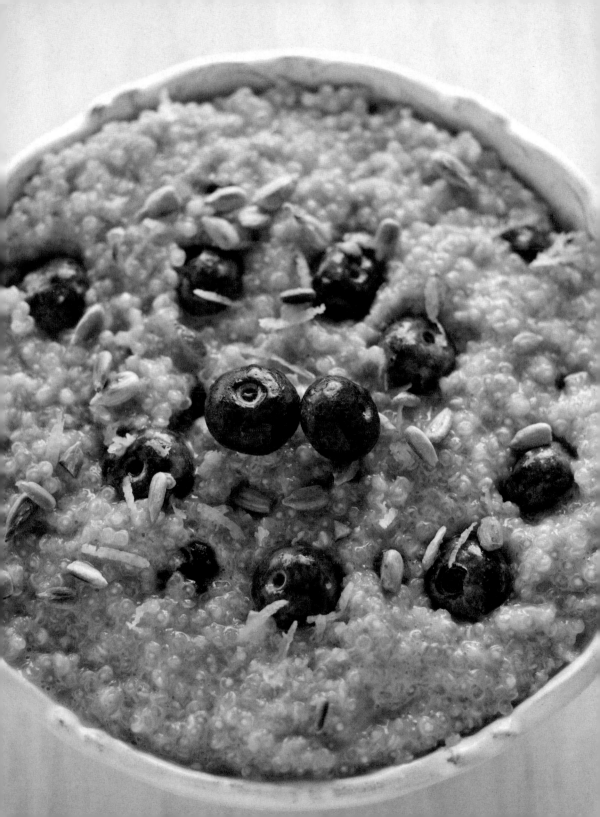

Broccoli-Quinoa *soup*

Vibrant and rich-tasting, this satisfying soup makes a delightful light lunch or dinner or a pleasing starter.

2 tablespoons **olive oil**

1 **onion**, finely chopped

1 cup **white quinoa, soaked, rinsed, and drained** (see page 38)

2 teaspoons minced **garlic**

7 cups **no-salt-added vegetable broth**

6 cups chopped **broccoli**

1 **russet potato**, peeled and chopped

2 tablespoons **raw or roasted cashew butter**

½ teaspoon **salt**

½ teaspoon **pepper**

Pinch **cayenne** (optional)

1 cup shredded **vegan or dairy Cheddar cheese**

Put the oil in a large soup pot over medium-high heat. Add the onion and cook, stirring frequently, until tender, for 10 to 12 minutes. Add the quinoa and garlic and cook, stirring constantly, for 1 to 2 minutes. Add the broth, broccoli, and potato. Increase the heat to high and bring to a boil. Decrease the heat to low, cover, and simmer until the quinoa is cooked and the potato is very soft, about 35 minutes.

Stir in the cashew butter, salt, pepper, and optional cayenne. Process with an immersion blender until smooth and creamy. Stir in the cheese until melted. Serve immediately.

46

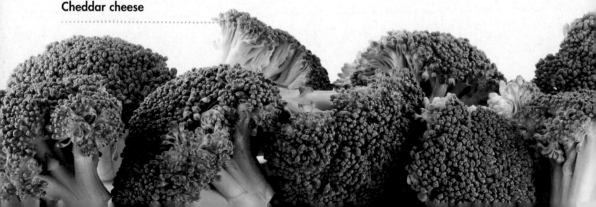

Spicy Quinoa-*carrot slaw*

This simple side dish comes together very quickly if you have cooked quinoa on hand in the refrigerator. For even faster prep, use bagged shredded carrots and break the speed limit.

2 cups cooked **quinoa** (see Basic Quinoa, page 42)

2 cups shredded **carrots**

½ cup chopped **fresh cilantro or parsley**

2 teaspoons **lemon zest** (optional)

3 tablespoons **extra-virgin olive oil**

3 tablespoons freshly squeezed **lemon or lime juice**

¼ teaspoon **cayenne**, plus more as desired

⅛ teaspoon **smoked paprika** (optional)

Put the quinoa, carrots, cilantro, and optional lemon zest in a medium bowl. Drizzle with the oil and lemon juice and sprinkle with the cayenne and optional paprika. Toss gently but thoroughly until well combined. Taste and add more cayenne if desired. Serve immediately or thoroughly chilled.

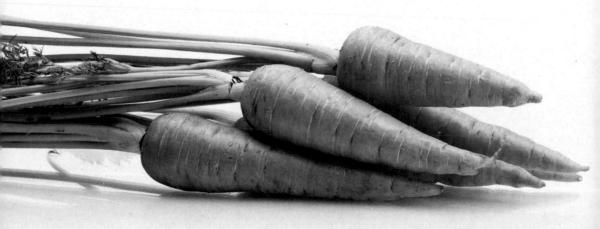

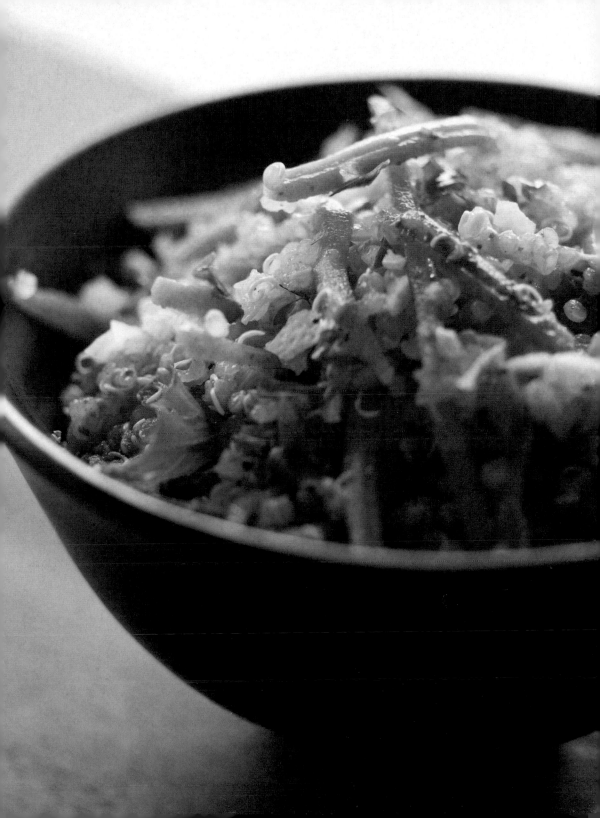

Quinoa with *spinach*

This vibrantly colored salad is bursting with flavor from the fresh herbs and vegetables.

5 cups stemmed **spinach, firmly** packed

¼ cup **fresh mint, basil, or cilantro leaves, firmly** packed

¼ cup **fresh parsley leaves,** firmly packed

¼ cup freshly squeezed **lemon juice**

¼ cup **extra-virgin olive oil**

2 tablespoons **reduced-sodium soy sauce**

4 cloves **garlic,** minced

2 cups cooked **quinoa** (see Basic Quinoa, page 42)

2 cups **grape tomatoes,** halved

1 cup peeled and diced **cucumber**

1 **green onion,** thinly sliced

Put the spinach, mint, and parsley in a food processor and pulse until chopped. Add the lemon juice, oil, soy sauce, and garlic and pulse just until well combined.

Put the quinoa, tomatoes, cucumber, and green onion in a large bowl. Add the spinach mixture and stir gently until evenly distributed. Serve immediately.

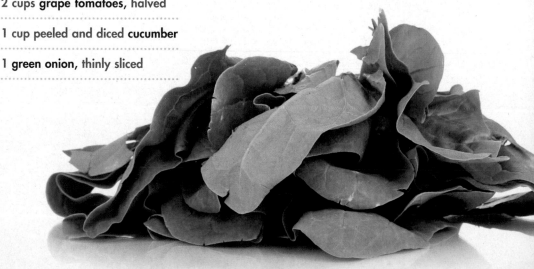

quinoa, bean, and avocado salad
with Creamy Lime Dressing

Quinoa and beans make a hearty, protein-rich combination, and the creamy lime dressing takes the flavors over the top.

CREAMY LIME DRESSING	SALAD
½ cup **vegan sour cream or nonfat plain Greek yogurt**	3 cups cooked **quinoa** (see Basic Quinoa, page 42)
3 tablespoons freshly squeezed **lime juice**	1 (15-ounce) can **no-salt-added red or black beans**, drained and rinsed
1 tablespoon chopped **fresh cilantro or parsley**	1 ripe **avocado**, diced
1 teaspoon **toasted sesame oil**	1 cup **grape tomatoes**, halved lengthwise
½ teaspoon **crushed red pepper flakes**	½ cup coarsely chopped **baby arugula, baby spinach, or fresh cilantro**, packed
Salt	
Freshly ground **pepper**	

To make the dressing, put the sour cream, lime juice, cilantro, oil, and red pepper flakes in a small bowl and whisk until well combined. Season with salt and pepper to taste and whisk again. If made in advance, store the dressing in the refrigerator for up to 5 days.

To make the salad, put the quinoa, beans, avocado, tomatoes, and arugula in a medium bowl. Add the dressing and toss gently until the salad ingredients and dressing are evenly distributed. Serve immediately, or chill for up to 4 hours before serving.

greek Quinoa

This showstopping dish has every color of the rainbow. It's a feast for the eyes and palate alike.

2½ cups **no-salt-added vegetable broth**

2 cups **quinoa, soaked, rinsed, and drained (see page 38)**

2 tablespoons **extra-virgin olive oil**

1 teaspoon **lemon zest**

2 teaspoons freshly squeezed **lemon juice**

1 teaspoon **rice wine vinegar**

1 teaspoon **dried mint**

½ teaspoon **salt**

1 cup **cherry tomatoes,** quartered

1 cup thinly sliced or shredded **red cabbage or radicchio**

½ cup diced **orange or yellow bell pepper**

½ cup diced **English cucumber**

½ cup finely diced or shredded **vegan cheese or crumbled feta cheese**

3 tablespoons chopped pitted **kalamata olives**

1 tablespoon minced **shallot** (optional)

Put the broth and quinoa in a large saucepan and bring to a boil over high heat. Decrease the heat to low, cover, and cook for 30 minutes. Remove from the heat and let sit, covered, for 5 minutes. Uncover and fluff with a fork. Let cool to room temperature.

Put the oil, lemon zest, lemon juice, vinegar, mint, and salt in a large bowl. Whisk until well combined. Add the quinoa, tomatoes, cabbage, bell pepper, cucumber, cheese, olives, and optional shallot and toss gently until evenly distributed. Serve immediately.

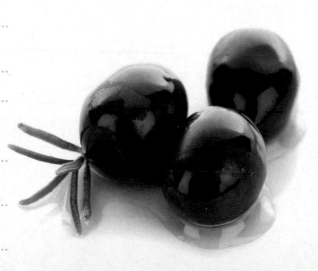

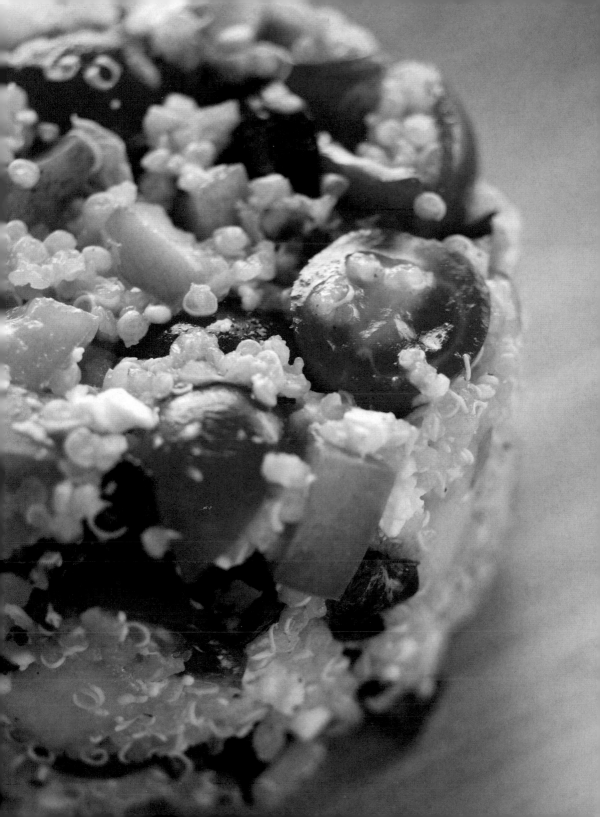

Thai-Inspired *quinoa salad*

Peanut butter makes everything taste great, including this mesmerizing combination of quinoa and crunchy raw vegetables.

4 tablespoons **no-salt-added smooth peanut butter**

4 tablespoons **seasoned rice wine vinegar**

2 tablespoons **reduced-sodium soy sauce**

½ teaspoon **crushed red pepper flakes**

1 small clove **garlic**, minced or pressed

2 tablespoons **hot water**, plus more if needed

3 cups cooked **quinoa** (see Basic Quinoa, page 42)

½ **English cucumber**, cut into julienne strips

1 **red bell pepper**, cut into julienne strips

1 small **carrot**, shredded or cut into julienne strips

1 cup shredded **red cabbage**

¼ cup chopped **fresh cilantro, mint, or basil**

¼ cup thinly sliced **scallions**

Put the peanut butter, vinegar, soy sauce, red pepper flakes, and garlic in a large bowl and mix well. Stir in the water to create a smooth sauce. If the mixture seems too thick, add up to 1 tablespoon of additional water, 1 teaspoon at a time, until the desired consistency is achieved. Add the quinoa, cucumber, bell pepper, carrot, cabbage, cilantro, and scallions and toss until evenly combined and the sauce is evenly distributed. Serve immediately or thoroughly chilled.

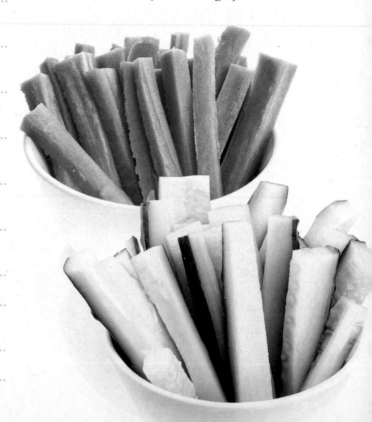

cheesy quinoa **and Broccoli Casserole**

This soothing, creamy casserole, featuring nutritious quinoa and broccoli, is comfort food at its finest.

3 cups cooked **quinoa** (see Basic Quinoa, page 42)

2 cups (16 ounces) **vegan sour cream or nonfat plain Greek yogurt**

2 cups shredded **vegan or dairy Cheddar cheese**

2 cups steamed **broccoli florets**

½ cup sliced **scallions**

½ cup shredded **carrot**

1 **jalapeño chile**, seeded and diced

1 teaspoon **ground cumin**

¼ teaspoon **salt** (optional)

¼ teaspoon **ground pepper**

Preheat oven to 350 degrees. Mist a 13 x 9-inch baking dish with cooking spray.

Put the quinoa, vegan sour cream, 1 cup of the cheese, and the broccoli, scallions, carrot, chile, cumin, optional salt, and pepper in a large bowl and mix well. Spoon into the prepared baking dish. Top with the remaining cup of cheese. Bake for 30 minutes. Serve hot.

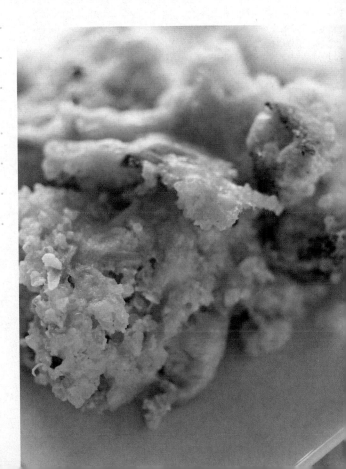

Quinoa *burgers*

Hearty and protein rich, these burgers combine three different forms of quinoa: the whole grain, flakes, and flour. With cooked quinoa on hand, they're a snap to prepare.

1 cup **cooked or canned chickpeas**, rinsed and drained

⅓ cup **quinoa flakes**

¼ cup chopped **onion**

1 clove of **garlic**, minced or pressed

1 cup cooked **quinoa** (see Basic Quinoa, page 42)

2 tablespoons **quinoa flour**, plus more if needed

2 tablespoons **water**, plus more if needed

1½ tablespoons **Italian seasoning blend**

¼ teaspoon **salt**

¼ teaspoon freshly ground **pepper**

Preheat the oven to 400 degrees F. Line a baking sheet with parchment paper.

Put the chickpeas, quinoa flakes, onion, and garlic in a food processor and pulse until the chickpeas are finely chopped but still have some texture. Transfer to a large bowl. Stir in the cooked quinoa, quinoa flour, water, Italian seasoning blend, salt, and pepper and mix well. The mixture should hold together when squeezed. If it's dry, add up to 2 tablespoons of additional water, 1 teaspoon at a time, until the mixture holds together. If it's too moist, add up to 2 more tablespoons of quinoa flour, 1 teaspoon at a time, until the mixture holds together.

Divide into four equal patties and arrange them on the prepared baking sheet. Bake for 10 minutes. Turn over and bake for 10 minutes longer.

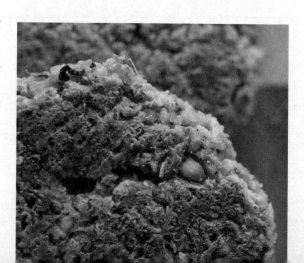

56

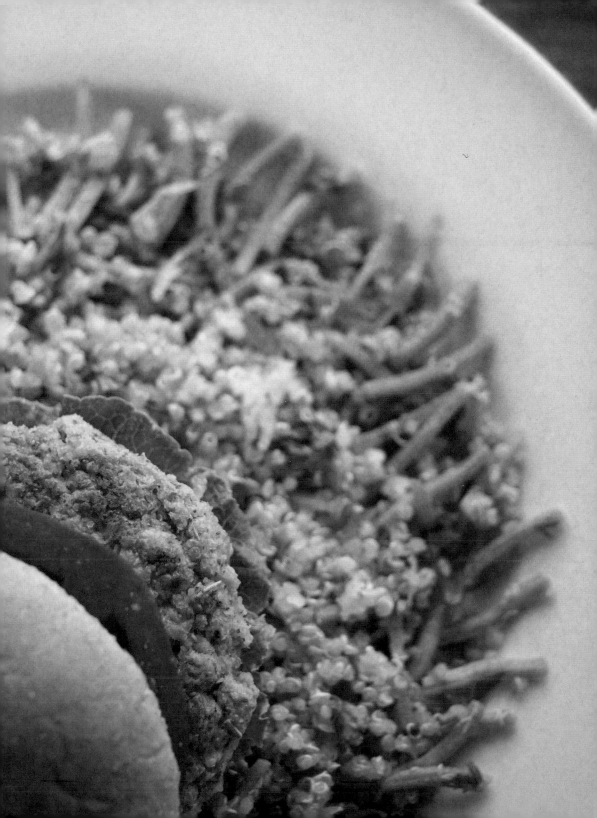

Mini Quinoa-*chocolate chip cakes*

Individual cakes, sweetened only with fruit, make a spectacular warm breakfast, satisfying dessert, or hunger-squelching treat any time of day.

2 cups **quinoa flakes**

1 cup **unsweetened applesauce**

¾ cup mashed **banana**

¼ cup **dairy-free chocolate chips**

¼ cup chopped **toasted pecans or walnuts**

Topping options: 4 teaspoons strawberry, cherry, or apricot jam; 4 teaspoons maple syrup; ½ cup fresh berries; ½ cup sliced fresh fruit (such as mango, peach, or banana)

Preheat the oven to 350 degrees F. Oil four oven-safe 16-ounce ramekins or baking dishes.

Put the quinoa flakes, applesauce, banana, chocolate chips, and pecans in a large bowl and mix until well combined. Spoon the mixture evenly into the prepared ramekins and smooth the tops. Bake for 25 to 30 minutes, until the cakes look firm and a toothpick inserted in the center comes out clean. Do not overbake. Cool in the ramekins for about 2 minutes, and then turn out onto individual plates. Serve hot or warm, garnished with the topping options of your choice.

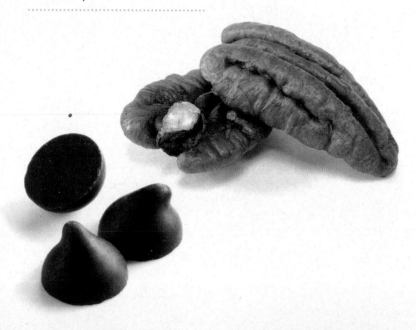

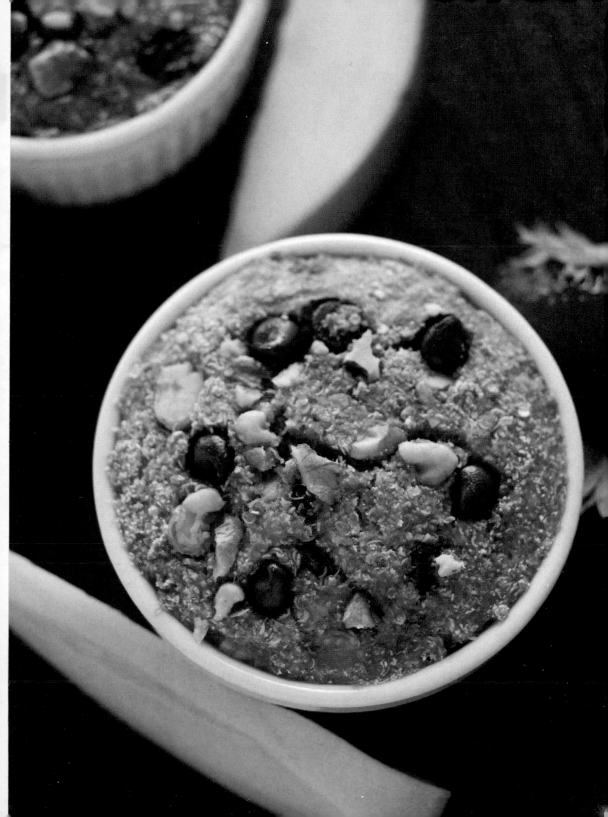

REFERENCES

Alvarez-Jubete, L., H. Wijngaard, E. Arendt, and E. Gallagher. 2010. "Polyphenol composition and in vitro antioxidant activity of amaranth, quinoa, buckwheat, and wheat as affected by sprouting and baking." *Food Chemistry* 119 (2):770–8.

Barclay, A., P. Petocz, J. McMillan-Price, V. Flood, T. Prvan, P. Mitchell, and J. Brand-Miller. 2008. "Glycemic index, glycemic load, and chronic disease risk: A meta-analysis of observational studies." *American Journal of Clinical Nutrition* 87:627–37.

Berti, C., P. Riso, A. Brusamolino, and M. Porrini. 2005. "Effect on appetite control of minor cereal and pseudocereal products." *British Journal of Nutrition* 94 (5):850–8.

Berti, C., P. Riso, and M. Porrini. 2004. "In vitro starch digestibility and in vivo glucose response of gluten-free foods and their gluten counterparts." *European Journal of Nutrition* 43 (4):198–204.

Lee, A., D. Ng, E. Dave, E. Ciaccio, and P. Green. 2009. "The effects of substituting alternative grains in the diet on the nutritional profile of the gluten-free diet." *Journal of Human Nutrition and Dietetics* 22 (4):359–63.

Mozaffarian, D., S. Kumanyika, R. Lemaitre, J. Olson, G. Burke, and D. Siscovick. 2003. "Cereal, fruit, and vegetable fiber intake and the risk of cardiovascular disease in elderly individuals." *Journal of the American Medical Association* 289 (13):1659–66.

Ranilla, L., E. Apostolidis, M. Genovese, F. Lajolo, and K. Shetty. 2009. "Evaluation of indigenous grains from the Peruvian region for antidiabetes and antihypertension potential using in vitro methods." *Journal of Medicinal Food* 12 (4):704–13.

Repo-Carrasco-Valencia, R., J. Hellstrom, J. Pihlava, and P. Mattila. 2010. "Flavonoids and other phenolic compounds in Andean indigenous grains: Quinoa (*Chenopodium quinoa*), kaniwa (*Chenopodium pallidicaule*) and kiwicha (*Amaranthus caudatus*)." *Food Chemistry* 120:128–133.

Rimm, E., A. Ascherio, E. Giovannucci, D. Spiegelman, M. Stampfer, and W. Willet. 1996. "Vegetable, fruit, and cereal fiber intake and risk of coronary heart disease among men." *Journal of the American Medical Association* 275 (6):447–51.

Saturni, L., G. Ferretti, and T. Bacchetti. 2010. "The Gluten-Free Diet: Safety and Nutritional Quality." *Nutrients* 2 (1):16–34.

Vega-Galvez, A., M. Miranda, J. Vergara, E. Uribe, L. Puente, and E. Martinez. 2010. "Nutrition facts and functional potential of quinoa (*Chenopodium quinoa* willd.), an ancient Andean grain: a review." *Journal of the Science of Food and Agriculture* 90 (15):2541–7.

Zevallos, V., H. Ellis, T. Suligol, L. Herencia, and P. Ciclitira. 2012. "Variable activation of immune response by quinoa (*Chenopodium quinoa* willd.) prolamins in celiac disease."*American Journal of Clinical Nutrition* 96 (2):337–44.

ABOUT THE AUTHOR

Beth Geisler is a writer and editor who specializes in the areas of food, health, and nutrition. She has been involved in alternative approaches to health and diet for more than a decade.

Jo Stepaniak is the author of more than a dozen books on vegetarian cooking and living, including *The Ultimate Uncheese Cookbook, Food Allergy Survival Guide,* and *Raising Vegetarian Children.*

© 2014 Beth Geisler and Jo Stepaniak

Photography: Andrew Schmidt, 123RF
Book design, photo editing: John Wincek
Editing: Beth Geisler, Jo Stepaniak

Pictured on front cover: Spicy Quinoa-Carrot Slaw, page 48

ISBN: 978-1-55312-050-6

Published by **Books Alive**
PO Box 99
Summertown, TN 38483
931-964-3571
888-260-8458
www.bookpubco.com

**books
Alive**

Printed in Hong Kong
Library of Congress Cataloging-in-Publication Data

Geisler, Beth.
    Quinoa : high protein, gluten free / Beth Geisler ; with recipes by Jo Stepaniak.
        pages cm
    Includes bibliographical references.
    ISBN 978-1-55312-050-6 (pbk.) — ISBN 978-1-55312-096-4 (e-book)
  1. Gluten-free diet—Recipes.   2. Quinoa.   3. Cooking (Quinoa)   I. Title.
    RM237.86.G45 2014
    641.3—dc23

                                                    2013035142

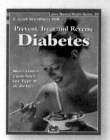
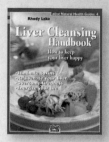
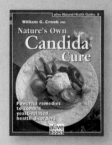
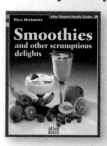
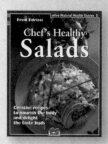
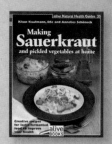
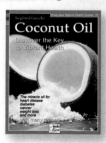
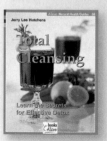
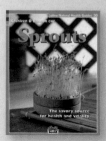
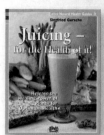
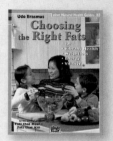
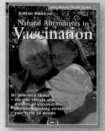